Generalized Anxiety Disorder

About the Authors

Craig D. Marker, PhD, is an Assistant Professor and Director of the Anxiety Research and Treatment Clinic at the University of Miami. His research interests focus on information processing in anxiety disorders, such as Generalized Anxiety Disorder and Social Anxiety Disorder.

Alison Aylward is currently a doctoral candidate in clinical psychology at the University of Miami. Her research interests include using an evolutionary approach to identify specific cognitive factors associated with various anxiety disorders such as Obsessive-Compulsive Disorder and Generalized Anxiety Disorder.

Advances in Psychotherapy – Evidence-Based Practice

Series Editor
Danny Wedding, PhD, MPH, Professor of Psychology, California School of Professional
    Psychology / Alliant International University, San Francisco, CA

Associate Editors
Larry Beutler, PhD, Professor, Palo Alto University / Pacific Graduate School of Psychology,
    Palo Alto, CA
Kenneth E. Freedland, PhD, Professor of Psychiatry and Psychology, Washington University
    School of Medicine, St. Louis, MO
Linda C. Sobell, PhD, ABPP, Professor, Center for Psychological Studies, Nova Southeastern
    University, Ft. Lauderdale, FL
David A. Wolfe, PhD, RBC Chair in Children's Mental Health, Centre for Addiction and Mental
    Health, University of Toronto, ON

The basic objective of this series is to provide therapists with practical, evidence-based treatment guidance for the most common disorders seen in clinical practice – and to do so in a "reader-friendly" manner. Each book in the series is both a compact "how-to-do" reference on a particular disorder for use by professional clinicians in their daily work, as well as an ideal educational resource for students and for practice-oriented continuing education.

The most important feature of the books is that they are practical and "reader-friendly:" All are structured similarly and all provide a compact and easy-to-follow guide to all aspects that are relevant in real-life practice. Tables, boxed clinical "pearls", marginal notes, and summary boxes assist orientation, while checklists provide tools for use in daily practice.

Generalized Anxiety Disorder

Craig D. Marker
Anxiety Research and Treatment Clinic, University of Miami, Coral Gables, FL

Alison G. Aylward
Department of Psychology, University of Miami, Coral Gables, FL

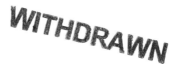

HOGREFE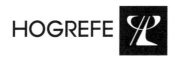

Library of Congress Cataloging in Publication

is available via the Library of Congress Marc Database under the
Library of Congress Control Number 2011933399

Library and Archives Canada Cataloguing in Publication

Marker, Craig D.
    Generalized anxiety disorder / Craig D. Marker, Alison G. Aylward.

(Advances in psychotherapy--evidence-based practice 24)
Includes bibliographical references.
ISBN 978-0-88937-335-8

    1. Anxiety disorders. I. Aylward, Alison G.
II. Title. III. Series: Advances in psychotherapy-- evidence-based practice ; 24

RC531.M37 2011   616.85'22   C2011-905071-4

PUBLISHING OFFICES
USA: Hogrefe Publishing, 875 Massachusetts Avenue, 7th Floor, Cambridge, MA 02139
                Phone (866) 823-4726, Fax (617) 354-6875; E-mail customerservice@hogrefe-publishing.co▮
EUROPE: Hogrefe Publishing, Merkelstr. 3, 37085 Göttingen, Germany
                Phone +49 551 99950-0, Fax +49 551 99950-425, E-mail publishing@hogrefe.com

SALES & DISTRIBUTION
USA: Hogrefe Publishing, Customer Services Department,
                30 Amberwood Parkway, Ashland, OH 44805
                Phone (800) 228-3749, Fax (419) 281-6883, E-mail customerservice@hogrefe.com
EUROPE: Hogrefe Publishing, Merkelstr. 3, 37085 Göttingen, Germany
                Phone +49 551 99950-0, Fax +49 551 99950-425, E-mail publishing@hogrefe.com

OTHER OFFICES
CANADA: Hogrefe Publishing, 660 Eglinton Ave. East, Suite 119-514, Toronto, Ontario, M4G 2K2
SWITZERLAND: Hogrefe Publishing, Länggass-Strasse 76, CH-3000 Bern 9

Hogrefe Publishing
Incorporated and registered in the Commonwealth of Massachusetts, USA, and in Göttingen, Lower Saxony,
Germany

Printed and bound in the USA
ISBN: 978-0-88937-335-8

Preface

Generalized anxiety disorder (GAD) refers to a condition in which someone has excessive worry that is uncontrollable. This disorder is one of the most common anxiety disorders; left untreated, it can lead to a significant impairment in a person's life. It is often a chronic condition, and it is associated with functional disability, poor quality of life, and increased health care costs (Borkovec & Ruscio, 2001). However, there are effective treatments for GAD, including psychological and pharmacological treatments. This book describes the components of an empirically supported psychological therapy for GAD. This treatment integrates components of cognitive techniques and exposure techniques, as well as newer techniques of mindfulness and acceptance practices. This book is intended for a variety of mental health professionals including psychologists, psychiatrists, social workers, general medical practitioners, other mental health professionals, and trainees in all of these fields.

> People with GAD experience uncontrollable worry about a range of topics

This book is divided into six chapters. The first two chapters are designed to provide a theoretical and descriptive overview of generalized anxiety disorder (GAD). Chapter 1 reviews prevalence, comorbidity, and differential diagnosis. GAD is often difficult to diagnose and some of the diagnostic confusion can be traced back to earlier diagnostic definitions that considered GAD a residual diagnosis if other anxiety disorders did not fit. The diagnosis of GAD is now much more reliable, and a reliable diagnosis is vital in treatment planning (Brown, Di Nardo, Lehman, & Campbell, 2001; Starcevic & Bogojevic, 1999). In Chapter 1, descriptions of common differential diagnoses are discussed in an attempt to assist the practitioner in providing the correct diagnosis. Chapter 2 reviews the leading theoretical models and research on the development and maintenance of GAD. Specifically, an attempt is made to discuss the most researched and theoretically relevant models, including intolerance of uncertainty, worry as cognitive avoidance, and positive beliefs about worrying.

Chapter 3 describes an overview of the key domains that should be considered when assessing someone with GAD. These domains are an important aspect of diagnosis. However, they are also vital to treatment in that the assessments can assist treatment planning in focusing on specific areas of difficulty. In Chapter 4, cognitive behavioral therapy (CBT) techniques for GAD are discussed. Each of these techniques is linked with theoretical models to provide a background of possible reasons each technique might work. Evidence on the efficacy of these techniques and practical suggestions for their application are also provided. Clinical descriptions are presented throughout the book, and Chapter 5 is dedicated to a clinical case vignette in which treatment is described from start to finish. Chapter 6 includes suggestions for further reading. The Appendix provides many useful assessment measures and clinical forms that can be utilized in treatment.

The empirical support for CBT for GAD is promising. This book attempts to bridge the divide between the research and day-to-day practice. Ideally, a practitioner will use this book with other readings, support from workshops and colleagues, and supervision opportunities.

Acknowledgments

This book is based on numerous experts' work on GAD, including that of Aaron T. Beck, Thomas D. Borkovec, Michel J. Dugas, Richard G. Heimberg, Robert Ladouceur, Colin MacLeod, Michael W. Otto, Susan M. Orsillo, Lizabeth Roemer, and many others.

We appreciate the numerous recommendations of Larry E. Beutler, who provided important editorial comments. We would also like to thank Robert Dimbleby of Hogrefe Publishing and series editor Danny Wedding for inviting us to participate in an important series on empirically supported therapies.

On a personal level, my development has been shaped by many mentors including Bethany A. Teachman, John E. Calamari, John L. Woodard, Peter J. Lang, Margaret M. Bradley, Linda C. Sobell, Mark B. Sobell, Jutta Joorman, John J. McArdle, and John R. Nesselroade. I would also like to thank Sarah who was responsible for much of my development as a writer. It was great to work with Alison on this project as she brought a fresh perspective and wonderful questions. I would like to thank my Mother, Father, and Sister for the loving support they provide. Finally, I would like to thank Viktoriya for her continued love, encouragement, support, and guidance.
CM

Many thanks to Craig Marker for the opportunity to work on this book. His trust in my abilities and his guidance have helped me to grow as a psychologist. I would also like to thank Debra Lieberman, Elaine Hatfield, and Alice F. Healy for their excellent mentorship. And finally, thanks to my family and friends for their unconditional love.
AA

Table of Contents

Preface v
Acknowledgments. vi

1   Description 1
1.1   Terminology 1
1.2   Definition 1
1.3   Epidemiology 3
1.4   Course and Prognosis 3
1.5   Differential Diagnosis. 4
1.5.1   Depression 4
1.5.2   Social Anxiety 5
1.5.3   Specific Phobia 5
1.5.4   Panic Disorder with Agoraphobia 5
1.5.5   Obsessive Compulsive Disorder. 6
1.5.6   Posttraumatic Stress Disorder. 6
1.6   Comorbidities 7
1.7   Diagnostic Procedures 7
1.7.1   Interviewer-Administered Measures 8
1.7.2   Self-Report Severity Measures 8
1.7.3   Assessing Suitability for Treatment 11

**2   Theories and Models of Generalized Anxiety
      Disorder** 12
2.1   Worry as Cognitive Avoidance 12
2.2   Positive Beliefs About Worry 14
2.3   Uncertainty and Worry 15
2.4   Information-Processing Biases Associated with GAD. 16
2.5   Metaworry 17
2.6   Implications for Treatment 18

3   Diagnosis and Treatment Indications 20
3.1   Key Features to be Assessed 20
3.1.1   Situational Triggers 20
3.1.2   Physical Features 21
3.1.3   Information Processing 21
3.1.4   Cognitive Avoidance Strategies 22
3.1.5   Intolerance of Uncertainty 22
3.1.6   Function of Worry. 22
3.1.7   Interpersonal Issues 23
3.1.8   Behavioral Avoidance. 23
3.1.9   Metaworry 23
3.1.10 Comorbidities 24
3.1.11 Functional Impairment 24
3.2   Overview of Effective Treatment Strategies 24

3.3   Factors that Influence Treatment Decisions 26
3.3.1   Age, Sex, and Ethnicity 26
3.3.2   Education 26
3.3.3   Family and Relationship Factors 27
3.3.4   Client Preference 27
3.3.5   Treatment History 27
3.3.6   Ability to Articulate Cognitions 27
3.3.7   Severity of Positive Beliefs About Worry 27
3.3.8   Comorbidities 28

4   Treatment 29
4.1   Methods of CBT 29
4.1.1   Psychoeducation 33
4.1.2   Cognitive Strategies 35
4.1.3   Exposure-Based Strategies 37
4.1.4   Relaxation and Acceptance-Based Strategies 40
4.2   Mechanisms of Action 41
4.2.1   Cognitive Models 41
4.2.2   Behavioral and Emotional Processing Models 42
4.2.3   Acceptance-Based Models 43
4.3   Efficacy and Prognosis 44
4.3.1   Efficacy of CBT 44
4.4   Combination Treatments 45
4.4.1   Medication Treatments 45
4.4.2   Comparing and Combining Medications and CBT 45
4.5   Overcoming Barriers to Treatment 45
4.5.1   Treatment Ambivalence 45
4.5.2   Homework Noncompliance 47
4.5.3   Adapting Treatment for Comorbidities 47
4.6   Adapting Treatment for Different Age Groups 48
4.6.1   Children and Adolescents 48
4.6.2   Older Adults 48
4.7   Adapting Treatment for Different Cultures 49

5   Case Vignette 50

6   Further Reading 57

7   References 58

8   Appendix: Tools and Resources 65

1

Description

1.1 Terminology

Generalized anxiety disorder (GAD) is characterized by excessive worry that is difficult to control. Worry is defined as an attempt to engage in mental problem solving on an uncertain issue with a potential threat outcome (Borkovec, Robinson, Pruzinsky, & Depree, 1983). GAD is diagnosed when the worry causes significant impairment and distress in the person's life, and it impairs the person's ability to function (e.g., at work or school, in relationships, etc.). Some common content areas of worry include:

- family/home/relationships
- finances
- work/school
- illness/health
- psychological/emotional
- future
- success/failure
- travel
- world issues
- minor matters.

The key difference between this diagnosis and "regular worry" is that the worry must be excessive (much more frequent than normal worry) and difficult for the person to control. The worries are not focused on one situation (e.g., having a panic attack or feeling embarrassed), but extend to a number of events.

1.2 Definition

GAD has undergone several changes within the last few editions of the *Diagnostic and Statistical Manual of Mental Disorders* (DSM; American Psychiatric Association, 1980, 1987, 1994). The term *GAD* first emerged with the publication of the DSM-III (American Psychiatric Association, 1980). At the time, GAD was described as "persistent anxiety," with symptoms of motor tension, autonomic hyperactivity, apprehensive expectation, and vigilance. The current *International Statistical Classification of Diseases and Related Health Problems* (ICD-10; World Health Organization, 1992) describes GAD in a very similar manner to the DSM-III, with generalized and persistent anxiety as the primary features. However, poor reliability of the DSM-III diagnosis of GAD was seen using these features. Also, GAD was seen as mainly a residual category for those patients who did not experience phobic avoidance or panic attacks. The DSM-III-R (American Psychiatric Association, 1987) improved upon the diagnostic criteria for GAD by shifting the primary feature from persistent anxiety to excessive or unrealistic worry (Starcevic & Bogojevic, 1999). The DSM-IV (American Psychiatric Association, 1994) further improved upon the definition of GAD and defined it as excessive worrying that is difficult to control (see Table 1). Thus, GAD is a chronic condition that is different from regular worry in that it is excessive (i.e., occurs with greater frequency than normal worry) and uncontrollable. Furthermore, a person with GAD must also endorse three or more of the following six symptoms: restlessness, fatigue, difficulty concentrating, irritability, muscle tension, or sleep disturbance. Another important feature is that the excessive worry must cause significant distress and impairment. The text revision of the DSM-IV (American Psychiatric Association, 2000) did not make any changes to the

Table 1.
DSM-IV-TR 300.02 Generalized Anxiety Disorder

A. Excessive anxiety and worry (apprehensive expectation), occurring more days than not for at least 6 months, about a number of events or activities (such as work or school performance).

B. The person finds it difficult to control the worry.

C. The anxiety and worry are associated with three (or more) of the following six symptoms (with at least some symptoms present for more days than not for the past 6 months). Note: Only one item is required in children.

(1) restlessness or feeling keyed up or on edge
(2) being easily fatigued
(3) difficulty concentrating or mind going blank
(4) irritability
(5) muscle tension
(6) sleep disturbance (difficulty falling or staying asleep, or restless unsatisfying sleep)

D. The focus of the anxiety and worry is not confined to features of an Axis I disorder, e.g., the anxiety or worry is not about having a Panic Attack (as in Panic Disorder), being embarrassed in public (as in Social Phobia), being contaminated (as in Obsessive-Compulsive Disorder), being away from home or close relatives (as in Separation Anxiety Disorder), gaining weight (as in Anorexia Nervosa), having multiple physical complaints (as in Somatization Disorder), or having a serious illness (as in Hypochondriasis), and the anxiety and worry do not occur exclusively during Posttraumatic Stress Disorder.

E. The anxiety, worry, or physical symptoms cause clinically significant distress or impairment in social, occupational, or other important areas of functioning.

F. The disturbance is not due to the direct physiological effects of a substance (e.g., a drug of abuse, a medication) or a general medical condition (e.g., hyperthyroidism) and does not occur exclusively during a Mood Disorder, a Psychotic Disorder, or a Pervasive Developmental Disorder.

diagnostic criteria. Furthermore, the proposed revisions to the DSM in the DSM-5 also do not make any revisions to the criteria (American Psychiatric Association, 2010).

1.3   Epidemiology

Previous differences in the definition of GAD make it difficult to investigate long-term data on prevalence and course of the disorder. However, starting with the DSM-III-R, there has been more consistency and reliability in the diagnosis of GAD. It has been estimated that in the course of 1 year, around 2% to 4% of the population will meet criteria for a diagnosis of GAD (National Comorbidity Survey; Wittchen, Zhao, Kessler, & Eaton, 1994). Over the course of a lifetime between 4% and 7% of the population will develop GAD at some point in their lives. In primary care facilities, GAD is the most likely anxiety disorder to be seen and the second most likely of all mental disorders (Barrett, Barrett, Oxman, & Gerber, 1988).

Lifetime incidence for GAD is between 4% and 7%

GAD seems to have a bimodal distribution in its age of onset. There are two age ranges when people are at greater risk for developing the disorder. The first period of risk occurs between the ages of 11 and the early 20s. There is also a late onset period where GAD develops in middle adulthood (Blazer, Hughes, & George, 1987; Brown, Barlow, & Liebowitz, 1994). GAD is more commonly seen among women than it is among men. In the general population, 4% of women were identified as having GAD, whereas 2% of men qualified for the diagnosis of GAD (National Comorbidity Survey; Wittchen et al., 1994).

1.4   Course and Prognosis

Patients in clinical studies (Mancuso, Townsend, & Mercante, 1993; Noyes, Holt, & Woodman, 1996) and participants of community epidemiological surveys (Blazer et al., 1991) retrospectively report that GAD is a chronic condition in which the episodes often last for a decade or longer. A prospective study of patients with anxiety followed patients for 5 years to observe the natural history of their disorders (Warshaw, Keller, & Stout, 1994; Yonkers, Massion, Warshaw, & Keller, 1996). Only 38% of people with GAD at baseline experienced a full remission at any time in the study. Thus, those with a history of GAD who also do not seek treatment seem to spend a significant proportion of their lifetimes with this disorder. Symptoms seem to wax and wane over time, but in general, the condition is chronic unless some form of treatment is received. For those individuals seeking treatment, cognitive behavioral therapy (CBT) seems to reduce the chronicity of this disorder. In one study (Borkovec & Costello, 1993), 57.9% of people treated with CBT techniques maintained those gains after 12 months (see Section 4.3 for more information on the efficacy of treatment).

GAD is unlikely to remit without treatment

1.5   Differential Diagnosis

It is common for GAD to coexist with other mental disorders

GAD has a high rate of comorbidity with many other disorders. Therefore, it is very important to rule in or rule out other potential disorders. This section provides information on which factors to attend to in order to differentiate the disorder from similar symptom patterns. It is recommended that clinicians use a semistructured interview such as the Structured Clinical Interview for DSM-IV (SCID-IV; First, Spitzer, Gibbon, & Williams, 2002) or the Anxiety Disorders Interview Schedule for DSM-IV (ADIS-IV; Brown, Di Nardo, & Barlow, 1994) to assess the presence of other Axis I disorders (see Section 1.7). Of note, two characteristics that have been found to accurately discriminate GAD from other disorders (but not necessarily from obsessive compulsive disorder [OCD]) are worry about worry (metaworry) and intolerance of uncertainty. Both of these constructs will be discussed in detail in Section 1.7.

Worry about worry and intolerance of uncertainty are specific to GAD

1.5.1   Depression

In GAD, negative thoughts most often focus on future threats; in depression, they reflect biased interpretations of self and world

At first glance, GAD and depression symptoms can present similarly, which can make a differential diagnosis tricky. For example, a common characteristic of both GAD and depression is the occurrence of repetitive negative thoughts. To make a differential diagnosis, one needs to examine the content and the time focus (past, present, or future) of these thoughts. Specifically, in depression, the content of negative thoughts is focused on pessimistic ideas about the self or world, with individuals experiencing repetitive negative thoughts about the past, known as rumination. In GAD, negative thoughts, known as worries, are more focused on future threats and how to deal with these threats. Thus one important differentiation between GAD and depression is whether the repetitive negative thoughts are better explained as ruminations (are the thoughts focused on negative aspects of the past?) or worries (are the negative thoughts focused on potential future threats?). It is also common for people with GAD and depression to have feelings of low self-worth or inadequacy.

Further questioning about the thoughts causing these feelings is helpful in making an appropriate diagnosis. For example, Diefenbach and colleagues (2001) found that people with GAD feel inadequate because they are more likely to focus their worries on loss of control, whereas people who are depressed feel inadequate because they ruminate about an aimless future. Likewise, on closer examination of these feelings of low self-worth, people with depression are more likely to have feelings of hopelessness, while people with GAD may be more likely to worry about their ability to cope and maintain control. Additionally, people with GAD are unlikely to experience these symptoms of depression: loss of interest in previously enjoyed activities, sadness, weight loss or weight gain, and recurrent thoughts about death. Likewise, people with depression will often not have the typical muscle tension seen in people with GAD. As seen in the Table 2, these disorders are highly comorbid, and it is likely that a client will have both disorders. Because of the chronic nature of GAD, depressive episodes are often interspersed within the course of GAD. A helpful assessment tool for measuring the symptoms and severity of depression is the Beck Depression Inventory 2 (BDI-II; Beck, Steer, & Brown, 1996). Higher scores indicate more severe depression symptoms (cutoffs: 0–13: minimal depression; 14–19: mild depression; 20–28: moderate depression; and 29–63: severe depression). The BDI-II has been shown to have good validity and reliability.

1.5.2   Social Anxiety

People with GAD, like people with social anxiety, may have excessive worries about relationships and performing in social situations. The main difference between these disorders is in how the fear or the worry is related to the social situation. People with social anxiety primarily fear how they will perform in social situations. That is, individuals with social anxiety are worried about negative evaluations of their performance, and they may worry about this performance before, during, and after an interpersonal interaction. This excessive fear causes individuals to avoid social situations where they may perform badly. While it is possible that people with GAD may have concerns about being evaluated negatively, these worries occur even when they are not performing or being evaluated. Moreover, these concerns are more likely one of many other (non-socially related) worries. For example, a person with GAD would likely worry about whether a relationship will work out, whereas a person with social anxiety might be more concerned with being embarrassed in front of his or her relationship partner (or saying something embarrassing). Also, the avoidance of feared situations that is seen in individuals with social anxiety is not common to individuals with GAD. Furthermore, people with social anxiety experience more psychophysiological arousal (e.g., sweating and blushing) than people with GAD experiences. If both diagnoses are to be given, then the social concerns by themselves must be significant enough to qualify for a diagnosis of social phobia. If there is little avoidance of social situations and the concerns seem to fit a larger picture of excessive worries, then a diagnosis of only GAD is more appropriate. A diagnostic interview (e.g., SCID-IV, ADIS-IV) may be sufficient to answer these questions.

1.5.3   Specific Phobia

Specific phobia is a fear of a particular stimulus (e.g., animals, heights, storms, blood, and airplanes). The fear is confined to that specific stimulus contrary to the general worry seen in GAD. Furthermore, a person with a specific phobia will have a large psychophysiological reaction in response to that feared stimulus (i.e., sweating, heart rate and respiration increase). A diagnostic interview may be sufficient to assess the presence of a specific phobia.

1.5.4   Panic Disorder with Agoraphobia

People with panic disorder mainly worry about having a panic attack. Although people with GAD may have panic attacks, a diagnosis of panic disorder requires that they have consistent worry about having a panic attack. In panic disorder, the worry or primary concern is confined to the physical symptoms, whereas in GAD, the worries are broad and range among many categories. Breitholz, Johansson, and Ost (1999) found that people with panic disorder have significantly more concerns about physical danger, whereas people with GAD are characterized by concerns about interpersonal conflicts and worry about significant others. In sum, if there is a history of panic attacks, one needs to assess if there is frequent worry about having another panic attack and if the worry focuses on somatic symptoms. If the client meets these criteria, then a diagnosis of Panic Disorder is appropriate. One can sufficiently assess these questions with a diagnostic interview.

1.5.5　Obsessive Compulsive Disorder

Worries reflect a broad range of real-life issues, whereas obsessions reflect specific types of intrusive thoughts

One difficulty in differentiating obsessive compulsive disorder (OCD) from GAD is that worrying and obsessing are often considered synonyms in our everyday language. Therefore, clients will often use these terms interchangeably. Although it is true that people with GAD and people with OCD experience negative thoughts, in OCD, these thoughts are upsetting and incongruent with the person's worldview (e.g., thoughts about stabbing someone with a knife). Additionally, these thoughts are intrusive and often lead to negative affect because of their disturbing nature. In contrast, in GAD, the thoughts are congruent with the person's worldview in that these thoughts or worries are about real-life circumstances (e.g., thoughts about a child's safety at school). These thoughts also lead to negative affect – not because of the thoughts themselves but rather through the amount of time spent worrying. For example, a persistent thought about finances is not an obsession, in terms of what constitutes an obsession in OCD, but rather a worry.

Another distinguishing factor between GAD and OCD is the possible range of thoughts experienced. For people with GAD, the client's worries can change quickly and vary widely. In contrast, a person with OCD has repeated, similar intrusive thoughts. Furthermore, a person with GAD does not use compulsions to get rid of worries, while a person with OCD will perform compulsive activities to minimize or eliminate his or her anxiety.

In sum, a diagnosis of GAD rather than OCD is appropriate when (1) the thoughts are worries, (2) the amount of time spent worrying is causing the negative affect, (3) the worries frequently change, and (4) compulsions are not used to relieve anxiety. However, if a diagnosis of OCD is suspected, the Yale-Brown Obsessive Compulsive Scale (Y-BOCS; Goodman et al, 1989a), a semistructured interview of symptoms specific to OCD, as well as one of the semistructured interviews mentioned above, can be administered to assess the presence of obsessions and compulsions.

1.5.6　Posttraumatic Stress Disorder

Posttraumatic stress disorder (PTSD) may be best characterized by anxiety related to the specific situation in which the trauma occurred and by symptoms of avoidance with regard to reminders of past traumatic events. Conversely, GAD is characterized by worry reactivity across a broad band of stimuli. Thus, if there is the presence of a trauma, and an individual's worry is specific to the trauma, a diagnosis of PTSD is appropriate. However, if there is a history of trauma, but the individual exhibits a broad range of worries that are both related and unrelated to the trauma, a diagnosis of both PTSD and GAD may be warranted. A diagnostic interview can be used to adequately assess the presence of this comorbidity.

1.6   Comorbidities

The section above describes differentiating GAD from other disorders. However, GAD commonly co-occurs with these same disorders. Thus, people are likely to have both GAD and one or more other disorders. In one study (Carter, Wittchen, Pfister, & Kessler, 2001), over 90% of people with GAD had at least one other diagnosis. Table 2 lists disorders that may be seen in association with GAD. Along with each disorder is the yearly incidence rate of that disorder for adults of the US population (National Institute of Mental Health, 2010). It is important to note that the percentages given for comorbidity represent the percentage of individuals with GAD who also have another disorder and not the percentage of individuals with a disorder other than GAD (e.g., depression) who also have GAD.

Table 2
Prevalence of Comorbid Disorders for Individuals with GAD

	Percentage of people with GAD and the listed disorder
Depression (6.7)*	59.0
Social Anxiety (6.8)	28.9
Specific Phobia (8.7)	29.3
Panic Disorder (2.7)	21.5
Obsessive Compulsive Disorder (1.0)	10.0
Posttraumatic Stress Disorder (3.5)	Not checked

Note. Generalized anxiety disorder (GAD) and depression are highly comorbid.
*Numbers in parentheses represent the incident rates per given year for the US population ages 18 and over.

1.7   Diagnostic Procedures

Accurate diagnosis of GAD is very important for selecting appropriate treatment methods. This section reviews the empirically established measures for assessing the presence and severity of GAD, as well as for documenting changes in these symptoms over the course of treatment.

1.7.1   Interviewer-Administered Measures

A structured
interview, SCID or
ADIS-IV, should be
administered at
the beginning of
treatment

There are two structured interviews that are commonly administered to diagnose GAD (based on DSM-IV-TR criteria) and common comorbid conditions. SCID-IV (First et al., 2002) and the ADIS-IV (Brown et al, 1994) both have good reliability and validity. The SCID can be found at www.scid4.org and the ADIS-IV is available from Oxford Press. We recommend you administer one of these structured interviews at the outset of treatment. As mentioned in Section 1.5, these interviews are helpful and often sufficient when making differential diagnoses.

1.7.2   Self-Report Severity Measures

It is important to measure multiple domains of GAD (e.g., intensity of worry, content of worry). These domains will be helpful in differential diagnosis, as well as in determining treatment focus. Many of these domains can be measured by self-report. Some potential targets of these domains are presented in Table 3. For a more thorough discussion of self-report measures, Antony, Orsillo, and Roemer (2001) provide useful resources on assessment of anxiety disorders. All measures discussed below are reproduced in the Appendix of the book.

Table 3
Targets of Self-Report Assessment in Generalized Anxiety Disorder (GAD)

	Measures
Intensity of worry	Penn State Worry Questionnaire
Content of worry	Worry Domains Questionnaire
Beliefs about worry (positive and negative)	Why Worry Scale Consequences of Worry Scale
Anxiety (cognitive and physiological)	Depression, Anxiety, and Stress Scale
Emotional avoidance	Acceptance and Action Questionnaire
Intolerance of uncertainty	Intolerance of Uncertainty Scale
Metaworry	Meta-Worry Questionnaire
GAD symptoms	Worry and Anxiety Questionnaire

Intensity of Worry

The PSWQ measures
intensity and
excessiveness of
pathological worry

Penn State Worry Questionnaire. The Penn State Worry Questionnaire (PSWQ; Meyer, Miller, Metzger, & Borkovec, 1990) is a 16-item self-report questionnaire that measures intensity and excessiveness of pathological worry without measuring content. The items are scored on a 5-point Likert scale (items 1, 3, 8, 10, and 11 are reverse scored; possible scores range from 16 to 80) with higher scores indicating higher severity of worry. Behar, Alcaine, Zuellig, and Borkovec (2003) found that a cutoff of 62 differentiated people with GAD from people with other anxiety disorders. This instrument was found to be a reliable and valid assessment of worry (Brown, Antony, & Barlow, 1992). The PSWQ is one of the most commonly used measures for assessing GAD. It is short, and the brevity of this tool allows it to be used frequently to measure treatment progress and outcome. This questionnaire is useful for assessing how much an individual worries; however, it does not provide information on the content of an individual's worries.

Content of Worry

Worry Domains Questionnaire. The Worry Domains Questionnaire (WDQ; Tallis, Eysenck, & Mathews, 1992) is a 25-item self-report measure that focuses on the content of worry by assessing 5 domains of worry: relationships (items 4, 16, 19, 21, 23), lack of confidence (items 2, 10, 15, 18, 20), aimless future (items 3, 5, 8, 13, 22), work (items 6, 14, 17, 24, 25), and financial concerns (items 1, 7, 9, 11, 12). The items are scored on a 5-point Likert scale (the range of each item is from 0 to 4). This measure has been found to have high test–retest reliability, as well as adequate validity (Stober, 1998) and internal consistency (Joormann & Stober, 1997). This measure is appropriate to use prior to beginning treatment to help illustrate the content of the person's worry. However, it is not well suited for diagnosis, as it was created with a nonclinical sample and does not differentiate well between individuals with and without GAD (Freeston, Rheaume, Letarte, Dugas, & Ladouceur, 1994). That said, this measure can be given following treatment to see if the breadth of an individual's worry has changed.

> The WDQ assesses the content of an individual's worry

Beliefs about Worry

Why Worry Scale. An important issue for treatment is to get an understanding of how an individual views worry (see also Section 2.2). The Why Worry Scale (WW-II; Freeston et al, 1994) measures the perceived positive consequences of worry and the reasons people engage in worry. It is a 25-item measure that assesses the following domains: aids in problem solving (items 3, 5, 9, 14, 21), motivates (items 8, 15, 16, 18, 19), protects from negative emotions in the event of a negative outcome (items 2, 4, 13, 22, 23), prevents negative outcomes (items 6, 11, 17, 20, 24), and worry as a positive personality trait (items 1, 7, 10, 12, 25). Each item is scored on a 5-point Likert scale (each item ranges from 1 to 5). The authors provide evidence that this measure is psychometrically sound, and individuals with GAD scored significantly higher on the scale than individuals who did not meet criteria for the disorder. This measure is best suited prior to beginning treatment to assess the positive value of worrying. It might also be used throughout treatment to assess change. However, it is not expected to change drastically during treatment, so it could be given less frequently than other GAD measures.

> The WW-II measures the perceived positive consequences of worry

Consequences of Worry Scale. The Consequences of Worry Scale (COWS; Davey, Tallis, & Capuzzo, 1996)measures the person's beliefs about the positive and negative consequences of their worry. It is a 29-item measure that has three negative consequences subscales: disrupting performance (items 1, 4, 5, 6, 12, 16, 23, 27), exaggerating the problem (items 11, 15, 18, 20, 26), and emotional distress (items 7, 10, 14, 19); it also has two positive consequence subscales: motivates (items 8, 9, 13, 22, 24, 29) and helps analytic thinking

> The COWS measures beliefs about the positive and negative consequences of worry

(items 2, 3, 17, 21, 25, 28). Each item is scored on a 5-point Likert scale (each item ranges from 1 to 5). The scale has been shown to have adequate reliability and validity (Covin, Dozois, & Westra, 2008; Davey et al, 1996). Similar to the WW-II, this measure is best suited to prior to beginning treatment to assess the value of worrying. It might also be used throughout treatment to assess change. However, it is not expected to change drastically during the course of treatment, so it can be given less frequently during treatment.

Anxiety

The DASS-21 measures depression, anxiety, and stress

Depression, Anxiety, and Stress Scale. The Depression, Anxiety, and Stress Scale (DASS-21; Lovibond & Lovibond, 1995; there is also a 42-item version) measures a person's depression (items 3, 5, 10, 13, 16, 17, 21), anxiety (items 2, 4, 7, 9, 15, 19, 20), and stress (items 1, 6, 8, 11, 12, 14, 18). The stress scale is characterized by nervous tension, difficulty relaxing, and irritability. It is thought to be related to GAD. However, all three subscales are moderately intercorrelated (r's between .5 and .7). Each item is scored on a 5-point Likert scale (each item ranges from 0 to 4). The overall measure has demonstrated psychometrically sound properties (Lovibond & Lovibond, 1995). This measure can be given very frequently throughout treatment to measure progress and treatment outcome.

Emotional Avoidance

The AAQ-II measures psychological flexibility and emotional avoidance

Acceptance and Action Questionnaire. People with GAD are thought to have higher amounts of emotional avoidance, and the Acceptance and Action Questionnaire (AAQ-II; Bond et al., 2011; Hayes et al., 2004) measures psychological flexibility and emotional avoidance. Although the AAQ-II might not discriminate GAD from other anxiety disorders, and while avoidance might be a common factor across anxiety disorders, it is still appropriate to measure this construct due to its importance in treatment. Items are scored on a 7-point Likert scale (range is from 10 to 70; each item is scored from 1 to 7; reverse score items 2, 3, 4, 5, 7, 8, and 9). The psychometric properties of this instrument are currently being examined (Bond et al, 2011). This measure is best suited for assessment prior to beginning treatment. It might also be used throughout treatment to assess change. However, the changes that occur on this measure are thought to be incremental, so the AAQ-II should be given less frequently throughout treatment.

Intolerance of Uncertainty

The IUS measures how much a person has difficulty tolerating uncertainty

Intolerance of Uncertainty Scale. The Intolerance of Uncertainty Scale (IUS; Freeston et al., 1994) measures how much a person has difficulty tolerating uncertainty, which has been associated with GAD (see also Section 2.3). It has 27 items that are scored on a 5-point Likert scale (range is from 27 to 135). Ladouceur and colleagues (2000) reported a mean of 87 ($SD = 21$) for a group diagnosed with GAD. The authors provide evidence that this measure is psychometrically sound and successfully discriminates between individuals with and without GAD (Dugas, Gagnon, Ladouceur, & Freeston, 1998; Ladouceur et al, 2000). Additionally, it predicts symptom severity among those with GAD (Dugas et al., 2007). This measure is best suited for assessment prior to beginning treatment, as well as assessing change in this possible predisposing factor.

If this measure is elevated following treatment, it might be a cause for concern due to the possibility for relapse.

Metaworry

Meta-Worry Questionnaire. The Meta-Worry Questionnaire (MWQ; Wells, 2005) is a 7-item questionnaire that measures beliefs about worry (see also Section 2.5). It is derived from the 65-item Meta-Cognitions Questionnaire (Cartwright-Hatton & Wells, 1997). The 7 items are scored on a 4-point Likert scale (range of each item is 1 to 4). This questionnaire has been found to be reliable and to discriminate worry in GAD from somatic anxiety, as well as to discriminate individuals with GAD from those with other disorders (Wells, 2005). This measure is best suited for assessment prior to beginning treatment. It might also be used to assess change in this potential predisposing factor.

GAD Symptoms

Worry and Anxiety Questionnaire. The Worry and Anxiety Questionnaire (WAQ; Dugas, Freeston, et al., 2001) is an 11-item questionnaire that assesses diagnostic criteria of GAD (based on the DSM-IV). Items are rated on a 9-point Likert scale (items range from 0 to 8). This measure may be suitable for a screening measure, but a clinical interview is warranted because the WAQ will often lead to false positives.

> **The WAQ is an 11-item questionnaire that assesses diagnostic criteria of GAD**

1.7.3 Assessing Suitability for Treatment

A person with GAD will typically have suffered with excessive worry for some time before seeking psychological treatment. Although this suffering provides great motivation to work on the symptoms of GAD, CBT requires that the client also be willing to engage in treatment and "buy into" the techniques. If someone has many positive beliefs about worry, then he or she might not be as willing to make changes to his or her worry as someone who has some negative beliefs about worry. As the CBT model is presented, the therapist should carefully assess the person's willingness to engage in treatment. One does not always expect the person to be fully ready for treatment. However, a person who expresses major concerns that the treatment will not work may be much more resistant to trying it. Assessment of the individual's previous attempts at dealing with the excessive worry is also important.

It is vitally important to maintain the client's motivation for treatment. A common technique used to enhance motivation is to have the client consider the disadvantages and advantages of continuing to use worry as a strategy. Because many people feel that there are positive benefits to their worry, it is also important to identify these benefits. However, listing the negative consequences will highlight the tremendous difficulties that come from the excessive worry.

2

Theories and Models of Generalized Anxiety Disorder

This chapter covers a number of models that have been proposed to explain how GAD, and more specifically worry, develops and how it is maintained. Each of these models has been substantially supported by research. These models cover three basic components of worry: predispositions to worry (one's intolerance of uncertainty and positive beliefs about worry), perceptions of threat (information-processing biases), and reinforcers of worry (worry as cognitive avoidance and metaworry). For the most part, these models are complimentary in that they can fit together within an overarching framework in which each model explains an important element in the origin or maintenance of excessive worry. This section presents the descriptions of each model followed by an attempt to integrate these models into one comprehensive model, which is presented at the end of the chapter. To illustrate these models, some case examples are included. Chapter 5 also includes a case vignette describing Laura, a 36-year-old mother of two, who was diagnosed with GAD.

2.1   Worry as Cognitive Avoidance

Tom Borkovec believes worry is a superficial mechanism that can be used to avoid deeper emotional content

One model of GAD, originally posited by Thomas Borkovec and colleagues, posits that worry is used as a means to avoid threatening cognitive and emotional content. Although this model may be counterintuitive at first, it posits that worry has an important function for people with GAD. Specifically, worry is thought to be a linguistic process that does not tap into deeper mental images (and thus anxiety related to these images). Thus, worrying does not allow deeper emotional processing. To say it another way, worry is used to avoid processing an emotional experience completely. Although the worry is troubling to the person with GAD, it may actually be serving as a way for the person to process negative information on a superficial level with less emotional intensity and distress. The person can avoid some of the negative emotions associated with the worry if he or she processes it only linguistically and without mental imagery. Indeed, studies have found that people who were worrying did not create imagery; rather worry was experienced as a negative verbal/linguistic activity (e.g., Borkovec & Inz, 1990). Additionally, Vrana, Cuthbert, and Lang (1986) found that people verbally articulating fear material created much less heart rate activity than when imagining the same frightening situation. Moreover, individuals have reported that they use worry to avoid more distressing topics (Borkovec & Roemer, 1995). Thus, worry is thought to only activate the verbal linguistic network and may be less distressing than other negative emotions.

In this model, worry is viewed as a negative reinforcer. Just as taking an aspirin gets rid of a headache, worry gets rid of negative emotions. Often, these negative emotions arise from a previous worry. Thus, the person may jump from worry to worry without fully processing any worry. In the short-term, the person feels relief from not experiencing the anxiety at a deeper level. However, in the long-term, worry inhibits the person from emotionally processing the information (see Figure 1). In addition, because of the reinforcement associated with worrying, the person may actually worry more. Thus, for people with GAD, worry is a paradox. The worry has short-term benefits of reducing negative emotion, but the worry has long-term consequences of causing greater distress. There is also some indication that people may be more susceptible to this process if they have greater intolerance for dealing with negative emotions. Thus, assessment of how one copes with negative emotions may also be important (see also the AAQ-II in the subsection "Emotional Avoidance" in Section 1.7.2). An important treatment implication stemming from this model is that a person with GAD may benefit from processing negative emotions more deeply to reduce levels of worry in the long-term (see also Section 4.1.3).

Worry helps people avoid experiencing negative emotions

Additionally, others have also highlighted that verbal processing impedes other environmental and experiential information from being processed (e.g., Roemer & Orsillo, 2002), which can prevent the learning of nonthreatening associations. Hayes, Strosahl, and Wilson (1999) purport that verbal processes initiate behavior through verbal contingencies rather than contact with contingencies that are present in the environment. Consequently, individuals may be relying on verbally rule-based behaviors while the environment presents contradictory information. Moreover, behavior that is verbally rule-based can be very resistant to disconfirming environmental evidence and will thus persevere (Hayes & Ju, 1998). As a result, worry prevents the extinction of fear because experiential avoidance is reinforced and the verbal-linguistic processes prevent experiential disconfirming associations from being learned.

Worry is a verbal process that prevents people from attending to important environmental information

For instance, let's consider a client, Mary, who came into treatment complaining of constant anxiety. She reports that she is "terrified of feeling anxiety" as soon as she wakes up in the morning and does "whatever I can to avoid it." She reports that she worries "all the time." And indeed, in session, she cannot seem to focus on detailing one worry but rather "jumps" from worry to worry. The therapist has a hard time focusing Mary because so many threatening worries are coming to her mind. When the therapist asks Mary if she ever focuses on the frightening images associated with one worry, she states, "I couldn't bear doing that" and "I avoid picturing anything related to my worries." Mary notices that she worries all the time, and she reports that she deliberately avoids focusing on the frightening images associated with her worry. Moreover, she feels that she is totally unable to control the constant worry she experiences. Mary's treatment will focus on helping her process these emotions more fully through the use of exposure (i.e., exposure to her worries).

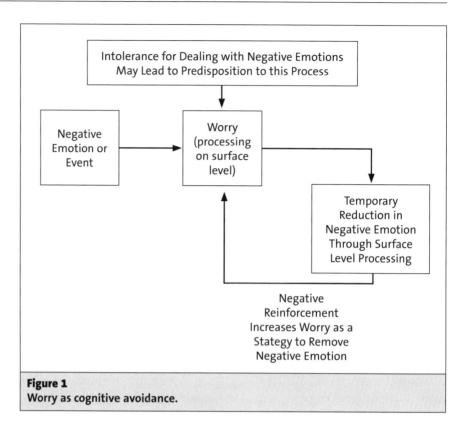

Figure 1
Worry as cognitive avoidance.

2.2   Positive Beliefs About Worry

Worry can help someone anticipate and plan for the future

Worry is thought by many people to have many positive qualities, such as aiding in anticipating and planning for bad outcomes in the future. For people with GAD, these positive qualities of worrying may be highly valued. People with GAD report that worry functions as a way to (1) avoid or prevent bad events, (2) motivate oneself to get things done, (3) prepare for the worst, (4) problem-solve, (5) distract oneself from even more emotional topics, and (6) superstitiously lessen the likelihood of bad events. Distracting oneself from more emotional topics coincides with the model of worry as an avoidance strategy (see above Section 2.1).

For people with GAD, their belief in the superstitious efficacy of worry is reinforced both by the nonoccurrence of feared outcomes and those situations in which they effectively deal with the stimuli triggering their worries. Consequently, their belief that worry is positive may be strengthened, and the frequency of worries may increase (see Figure 2). However, recent research has found that inducing positive beliefs about worry does not necessarily lead to more worry (Prados, 2010). That said, this research was done on a nonclinical population, and the results may not generalize to individuals with GAD. Therefore, it is recommended that changing these beliefs be an important component of CBT (see Section 4.1.2).

For example, Mary expressed that she "has to" worry because otherwise she would not effectively handle important situations. She reports that if she

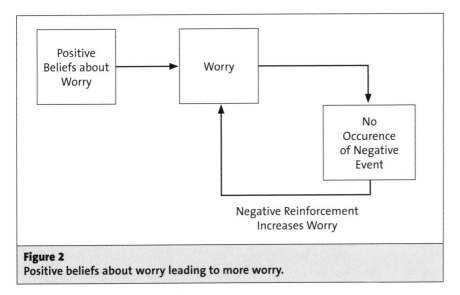

Figure 2
Positive beliefs about worry leading to more worry.

stopped worrying, she would not be doing all she could to avoid negative consequences. She remembers that worry has helped her plan for difficult situations in the past (e.g., taking final exams). The therapist's role is to address this overvaluation of worry by helping the client investigate the pros and cons associated with using worry in this manner. That is, motivational interviewing techniques can be used to determine how useful worry is in the context of the negative consequences that are caused by excessive worry.

2.3   Uncertainty and Worry

Individuals with intolerance of uncertainty believe that uncertainty should be avoided, and they experience uncertainty as highly distressing. Michel Dugas, Robert Ladouceur and their colleagues are responsible for much of the literature on intolerance of uncertainty and its implications for GAD. For example, their research has shown that people with GAD find it more difficult to tolerate and accept uncertainty than people without GAD (Dugas et al., 1998). They believe that this intolerance is a predisposing factor for developing GAD (much the same way that anxiety sensitivity is thought to be a predisposing factor for panic disorder). For people with GAD, there is often a need for certainty in order to not worry. If they do not feel complete certainty, then they might engage in worry to deal with the distress of this uncertainty. That is, worry might be an ineffective attempt to control and reduce uncertainty (see Figure 3). Thus, worry is again reinforced because it reduces the negative affect associated with intolerance of uncertainty. In fact, experimental evidence shows that increasing intolerance of uncertainty led to increases in worry (Ladouceur et al., 2000), corroborating the causal role of this trait on worry. Moreover, as mentioned earlier, intolerance of uncertainty has been found to be specific to GAD compared with other anxiety disorders (but not necessarily OCD; Dugas, Marchand, & Ladouceur, 2005; Ladouceur et al., 1999) and predicts symptom severity among those with GAD (Dugas et al., 2007).

Individuals who experience distress in the face of uncertainty use worry to gain more certainty

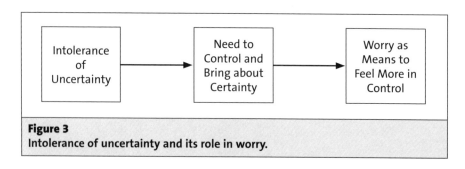

Figure 3
Intolerance of uncertainty and its role in worry.

The client described earlier, Mary, demonstrates a marked intolerance of uncertainty in session. She continually seeks reassurance from the therapist that "everything is going to be OK." In addition, she admits that she is constantly asking others how they think certain things in her life will turn out. Even though everybody tells her either that they do not know or that she will find out eventually, she says she "hates not knowing the answer now." For example, Mary is pregnant, and she worries that her constant anxiety will hurt her baby as well as predispose her to getting postpartum depression. She makes frequent calls and visits to her doctor's office to get his reassurance. Even though the doctor assures her that the baby is healthy and that Mary will be fine, she continually worries and continues to seek reassurance because she does not know for certain. These strategies that Mary uses to deal with the uncertainties in her life are addressed in treatment.

2.4   Information-Processing Biases Associated with GAD

The way that people process information from the environment is thought to play an important role in the development and maintenance of anxiety disorders. One processing bias seen in people with GAD is an attention bias for threat. That is, people with GAD may be scanning the environment in a way in which they are quick to perceive threat or slow to disengage from threat (see Mogg & Bradley, 2005, for a review of the literature on this topic). For example, many studies have demonstrated this attention bias for threatening words (related to worries) and threatening pictures. Moreover, there is evidence that engaging with threatening meanings (i.e., attending to threat and processing its meaning) leads to an increase in worry (Hirsch et al., 2010). Thus, a person with GAD might be hypervigilant in detecting particular threats, which may lead to worry.

People with GAD may interpret ambiguous stimuli as threatening

Another bias that may be common among people with GAD is an interpretation bias. That is, people with GAD may interpret ambiguous stimuli as threatening and thus see these stimuli as leading to negative outcomes (Eysenck, MacLeod, & Mathews, 1987; Eysenck, Mogg, May, Richards, & Mathews, 1991; Mathews, Richards, & Eysenck, 1989; Mogg, Bradley, Miller, & Potts, 1994). For example, people with GAD may watch the news and interpret events as being more personally threatening than those events would be to others watching the same broadcast. Additionally, individuals with GAD

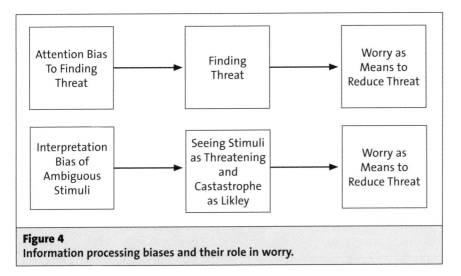

Figure 4
Information processing biases and their role in worry.

have been found to make catastrophic predictions about events that have a low probability of occurring (Borkovec, Shadick, & Hopkins, 1991; Butler & Matthews, 1987; Dugas et al., 1998). That is, they overestimate the magnitude of the feared outcome as well as the likelihood that the outcome will occur. The combination of an attention bias (which may lead people with GAD to attend to more threats) and an interpretation bias (which may lead to more negative and threatening interpretations of events) can lead to exacerbation of GAD symptoms (see Figure 4).

As an example, Mary reports noticing things on the news or the Internet and thinking that her baby or family is in danger. For example, any time she hears about a crime on the news, she worries that her husband has been hurt and calls him repeatedly until she finds out he is safe. As well, whenever she hears about a problem pregnancy, she worries that she will experience the same problem. Similarly, she interprets any ambiguous bodily sensations as issues with her baby's health. In short, she is hyperattentive to dangers and thus misinterprets safe situations as harmful.

People with GAD display both an attention bias and an interpretation bias

2.5   Metaworry

Adrian Wells and Gerald Matthews are largely responsible for the model of metaworry. Metaworry is basically worry about worry. Specifically, for people with GAD, there is often a belief that worry is associated with going crazy or that worry is uncontrollable. Thus, these individuals start to worry about how much they are worrying (see Figure 5), and worry itself becomes a focus of the person's worries. This factor has been found to be a good discriminator between GAD and other anxiety disorders (but not necessarily OCD).

When asked about how she feels about worry, Mary reported that she is "afraid" of how much she worries. She said that as soon as she wakes up in the morning, she fears when the worry will start again. In fact, one of her worries is that she is going to "go crazy with worry" because she feels that the worry is "completely out of my control."

Metaworry is basically worry about worry

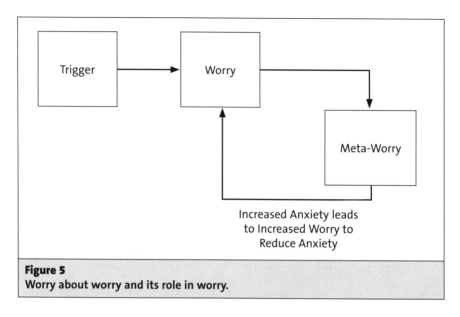

Figure 5
Worry about worry and its role in worry.

2.6   Implications for Treatment

Treatment for GAD attempts to include all aspects of the above models of GAD. Figure 6 integrates the different models into one diagram. Predisposing factors such as intolerance of uncertainty and positive beliefs of worry may make a person more prone to worry. Information-processing differences (i.e.,

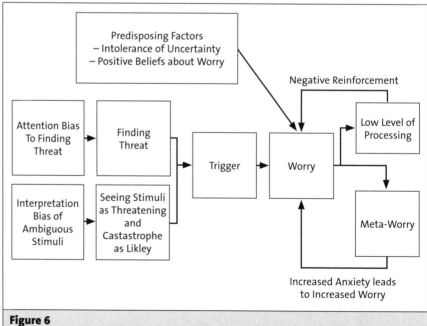

Figure 6
Comprehensive model of factors associated with generalized anxiety disorder (GAD).

attention bias and interpretation bias) may lead the person to find more threat in the environment and interpret ambiguous stimuli as more threatening. As a strategy to reduce the negative emotions associated with these threats, the person processes information on a superficial linguistic level (without fully processing it more deeply). This strategy is negatively reinforced because it temporarily reduces distress. Thus, worry becomes a process to avoid negative emotions.

During CBT, therapists attempt to reduce this low level of processing by having clients "worry out" their negative emotions. That is, exposure therapy allows individuals to process the worry on a deeper level to help them realize that they can cope with their negative emotions. Of note, although GAD is mostly characterized by the aforementioned cognitive avoidance, behavioral avoidance of situations (e.g., social situations) is seen in over half of individuals with GAD (Butler, Gelder, Hibbert, Cullington, & Klimes, 1987) and will be important to address with exposure therapy. Cognitive therapy attempts to help individuals reevaluate (1) the positive benefits of worrying, (2) interpretation biases of ambiguous stimuli, (3) their intolerance of uncertainty, and (4) their metaworry. Furthermore, acceptance-based strategies and relaxation strategies help clients deal with both uncertainty and the muscle tension associated with worry.

Diagnosis and Treatment Indications

This chapter provides the clinician with a framework for understanding a client's GAD and for selecting an appropriate course of treatment. It begins with a discussion of key features to be assessed, followed by an overview of effective treatment strategies and guidelines on how to use information from the assessment to help guide a plan for treatment.

3.1   Key Features to be Assessed

Key features that should be assessed include situational triggers, physical features, information processing, cognitive avoidance strategies, intolerance of uncertainty, beliefs about the function of worry, interpersonal issues, behavioral avoidance, and metaworry. The extent that these various features are present will influence the type of strategies that are used. Many of the instruments that are mentioned to assess these features are discussed in Chapter 1 and are available in the Appendices.

3.1.1   Situational Triggers

GAD presents itself differently than other anxiety disorders in regards to situational triggers. In specific phobia or social anxiety, there is a clear identifying situational trigger that brings about fear, and this trigger is often avoided. However, triggers for worries can come from many sources. A careful assessment of situational triggers would include asking questions such as those below.

Questions to Ask

"In what situations do you notice yourself worrying more?"

"In what situations do you find yourself worrying less?"

"Does anything you do lead to more (or less) worrying?"

"Can you control your worries?"

"When do worries come into your mind for no apparent reason?"

In GAD, situational triggers are more diffuse and may be harder to identify than in other anxiety disorders

Knowing when the client's worry is worse and what helps lessen the worry has important therapeutic implications. These situational triggers may aid in determining which strategies will be helpful in reducing the client's worry.

3.1.2 Physical Features

GAD presents a different physiological profile than other anxiety disorders. Although people with GAD may have panic attacks, the physiological symptoms related to fear might not be commonly experienced in those with GAD as they are in other anxiety disorders. People with GAD do, however, often experience a great deal of muscle tension from worrying over a long period. Muscle tension is unique to GAD, and it is not a diagnostic criterion for other anxiety disorders or depression. Although one could provide a comprehensive electromyography exam to assess muscle tension, a self-report of where and when muscle tension is commonly felt is usually sufficient.

The experience of muscle tension is only seen in GAD

3.1.3 Information Processing

As mentioned in Section 2.4, people with GAD often process ambiguous stimuli as threatening. More specifically, this might mean that people with GAD will worry about things that other people do not perceive as threatening. Some examples include worrying about minor matters or world events. One study (Barlow, 1988) found that the question "Do you worry excessively about minor things?" effectively discriminated individuals with GAD from other disorders. Furthermore, another study by Roemer, Molina, and Borkovec (1997) found that minor matters was a category of worry that people with GAD endorsed significantly more often than a nonclinical group (see Table 4).

Patients with GAD worry about relatively minor matters

Table 4
Content of Worries (Percentages of Worries)

Subject of Worries	GAD	Nonclinical
Family/Home/Relationships	31.4	28.2
Work/School	22.0	36.6
Illness/Health	9.6	9.9
Finances	10.8	5.6
Miscellaneous (subcategories below)	26.3	19.7
Success/Failure	14.8	35.7
Future	12.2	14.3
Psychological/Emotional	20.9	28.6
Minor Matters / Routine	45.2	7.1
Travel	6.9	14.3

Note. GAD = generalized anxiety disorder. Adapted from Roemer, Molina, Litz, & Borkovec (1997).

Thus, some questions that might assess the negative interpretation of ambiguous stimuli could include:

- "Do you find that you worry excessively about minor matters (such as punctuality, household tasks, and repairs)? That is, do you worry about the 'small stuff'?"
- "Do you worry about world events or things you see on the news?"

3.1.4   Cognitive Avoidance Strategies

People with GAD may use worry to avoid deeper processing of negative emotions

As noted in Section 2.1, people with GAD may use worry as a way to avoid deeper processing of negative emotions. Thus, they may jump from worry to worry. It is important to assess how much a person engages in this cognitive avoidance strategy. A possible question to ask is "Do you find yourself jumping from worry to worry?"

Self-report measures of the intensity of worry (see the subsection "Intensity of Worry" in Section 1.7.2) and GAD symptoms (see the subsection "GAD Symptoms" in Section 1.7.2) may predict how easy it is for a person to control his or her worry. It might be that the person cannot control his or her worries because he or she is jumping from worry to worry. Knowing how much people jump from worry to worry will be important when designing "worry exposures," in which the person will fully process the worry (see Section 4.1.3).

3.1.5   Intolerance of Uncertainty

Intolerance of uncertainty is a feature of GAD that might be vital for the development and maintenance of GAD. It is thought to be a predispositional factor in that people who cannot tolerate uncertainty may engage in behaviors (e.g., worry) in the hopes of gaining more certainty. The IUS (see the subsection "Intolerance of Uncertainty" in Section 1.7.2, and the Appendix) is an excellent measure to assess a person's comfort with uncertainty. Additional follow-up on this questionnaire can be helpful in assessing this very important construct and planning therapeutic interventions.

3.1.6   Function of Worry

If intolerance of uncertainty is a predisposing factor for GAD, then positive beliefs about worry might be the causal link between intolerance of uncertainty and worry. That is, a person who is distressed about uncertainty may worry to lower this distress. But, if this person does not believe that worry will help relieve the distress, then the causal chain is broken (however, one study did not find evidence for this causal chain; see Prados, 2010). Thus, it is important to find out how much a person believes that worry is useful. In therapy, this knowledge will translate into cognitive restructuring strategies to assess the short- and long-term benefits of worry and help the client and therapist weigh the pros and cons of worry.

3.1.7   Interpersonal Issues

People with GAD often have frequent occurrences of interpersonal worries about relationships. Furthermore, Borkovec and colleagues (e.g., Borkovec, Newman, & Castonguay, 2004) found that interpersonal issues were common in GAD. For example, people with GAD may have patterns of enmeshment with other family members. This pattern may need to be considered in the course of treatment. To assess interpersonal issues, the Inventory of Interpersonal Problems Circumplex Scales (Alden, Wiggins, & Pincus, 1990) may be useful. The treatment outlined in this book does not emphasize these potential issues. However, if significant issues are found, interventions that include family members (if possible) may be helpful. There have been a number of recent interventions focusing on family-based CBT for children (see Barmish & Kendall, 2005; Ginsburg & Schlossberg, 2002), but more research is needed to study the benefit of bringing in family members when treating adults with anxiety. If a practitioner decides to bring in family members, there are many potential issues to consider, including: (1) the supportiveness of family members for the client's changing (and hence changing their relationship), (2) the benefits for the family member if the client stays the same (the family member may benefit in some way from the clients current state), and (3) whether the family member can change his or her behavior (often he or she may have been in a long-standing pattern of relating to the client, which can be difficult to change).

3.1.8   Behavioral Avoidance

Some clients may engage in avoidance of situations, or they may use safety behaviors to reduce the distress associated with worry. Likewise, reassurance seeking can be thought of as a safety behavior that is intended to increase certainty (and thus to avoid the distress of uncertainty). For example, a client may continually call her husband to make sure he is all right. It will be important to create exposures to these fears so that the avoidance and safety behaviors can be treated (e.g., having the client challenge herself to not call her husband numerous times during the day). Similarly, clients may be avoiding certain situations because these situations can lead to more worry (e.g., being out of cell phone reach when a child is not home). Again, a list of all relevant avoidant and safety behaviors will be needed later in treatment to help the client learn to tolerate uncertainty. Questions the therapist might ask include the following:

- "Is there anything you do to reassure yourself when you are worried about something?"
- "Are there any situations you avoid because you are worried something will happen?"

People with GAD often seek reassurance from others to gain certainty and to avoid distress

3.1.9   Metaworry

The presence of worrying about worry (or metaworry) is a good differential tool that can help the clinician decide whether a person has normal or exces-

Simply asking "Do you worry about how much you are worrying?" will help differentiate GAD from other anxiety disorders

sive worry. A simple question such as "Do you worry about how much you are worrying?" may be enough to assess metaworry, and it can differentiate GAD from other anxiety disorders. However, the 7-item MWQ (see the subsection "Metaworry" in Section 1.7.2) is a more sophisticated tool to assess worry about worry. As described in Section 2.5, metaworry might lead to a person feeling more distress. Thus, it is important to determine how metaworry is affecting the person's worry cycle. It is also important to determine whether some of the therapeutic cognitive strategies should be implemented to determine the pros and cons of these thoughts.

3.1.10 Comorbidities

It is important to assess the degree of comorbidity and the relative severity of each comorbid condition prior to treatment. Furthermore, it should also be assessed whether comorbid problems are likely to interfere with the treatment of GAD. For example, severe depression might need to be treated prior to engaging in the treatment of GAD. The structured clinical interviews (ADIS-IV or SCID-IV; see Section 1.7.1) are a way to assess for comorbid conditions. Likewise, the Psychiatric Diagnostic Screening Questionnaire (Zimmerman & Mattia, 2001a, 2001b), a 125-item self-report measure, assesses the patient's standing on 13 different DSM-IV Axis I categories.

3.1.11 Functional Impairment

It is critical to assess daily functioning in GAD patients

Assessing impairment in the person's daily functioning is important for many reasons. One reason is that the degree of functional impairment may influence treatment. That is, individuals who feel that they worry a great deal but do not experience functional impairment may not qualify for a diagnosis of GAD and may not need treatment. If the degree of impairment is severe enough that the person is unable to function at work or has interpersonal problems, then focus on these other areas is also important in treatment.

3.2 Overview of Effective Treatment Strategies

Effective treatment for GAD should aim to change biased cognitions, avoidance of distress, and intolerance of uncertainty

The most frequently studied, evidenced-based, psychological strategies for treating GAD include (1) cognitive strategies, (2) exposure-based strategies, and (3) acceptance-based strategies. Each of these is described in Table 5. Evidence-based psychological treatments for GAD usually include various combinations of cognitive, exposure, and acceptance strategies. Together these strategies comprise a comprehensive CBT intervention for treating GAD. Different studies have employed and studied the impact of the different components of these therapies, and we do not know which components are the most important within a comprehensive program of treatment (see Behar, DiMarco, Hekler, Mohlman, & Staples, 2009, or Borkovec, Newman, Pincus, & Lytle, 2002). What is clear is that the combination of these components is effective.

Pharmacological Treatments for GAD

Benzodiazepines

Compared with placebo, benzodiazepines provide GAD sufferers with effective and rapid symptomatic relief over the short term. They are quick–acting and reduce anxiety symptoms. Despite these advantages, there is agreement that they are not appropriate as treatment for a chronic condition and should be used for no more than 2–4 weeks. In general, the short-term benefits are outweighed by the problems associated with dependency, sedation, and increased risks of neonatal and infant mortality when used in late pregnancy or while breastfeeding. A substantial proportion of individuals develop rebound anxiety, an intensification of previous symptoms, or a withdrawal syndrome when treatment with benzodiazepines is discontinued.

Buspirone

Buspirone once held considerable promise as a successor to benzodiazepine treatment because it was nonsedating and did not produce dependence. However, its anxiolytic effects appear to be somewhat less than benzodiazepines, particularly with more severe anxiety, and recent reviews provide only equivocal evidence for its superiority over placebo. Potential disadvantages include a lag of several weeks before symptom relief occurs and possible dysphoric side effects.

Antidepressants

Clinical guidelines recommend antidepressants, principally selective serotonin reuptake inhibitors (SSRIs; e.g., escitalopram, paroxetine, sertraline), as treatment for GAD on the grounds of safety, tolerability, and effectiveness. This class of medication is also effective with the comorbid conditions that are common in GAD, such as depression. Studies of the long-term efficacy of antidepressants, with follow-up periods of years rather than months, have yet to be conducted. Efficacy over 6-month follow-up periods has recently been studied with GAD patients. Greater remission rates than placebo were found at 6 months (69% versus 42–46%).

In addition to psychological approaches for treating GAD, there is evidence supporting pharmacological treatments. Reasonable numbers of large randomized placebo-controlled trials with GAD have been conducted with three classes of pharmacotherapy. The basic medications and descriptions are listed below.

Table 5
Evidence-Based Psychological Strategies for Treating GAD

Treatment strategy	Description
Cognitive	• Weighs pros and cons of the positive value of worry (helps the person decide whether worry is actually helpful, or whether the extreme worry leads to more difficulties than it helps). Additionally, cognitive therapy can assist in weighing the pros and cons of whether worrying about how much the person worries (metaworry) is actually a helpful thought.

Table 5 (continued)

	• Assists in determining whether ambiguous stimuli (e.g., a news broadcast) are actually as risky or as catastrophic as the person believes (i.e., reassess the risk of stimuli, to provide a more accurate risk assessment, and reassess the likely outcome to provide a more accurate picture of the situation). • Involves helping the client determine how important it is to be certain (i.e., evaluating intolerance of uncertainty), and whether it is valuable to keep this belief.
Exposure	• Assists the client in fully emotionally processing negative emotions rather than viewing them on a surface level (as in worry). • Assists the client in seeing that he or she can deal with negative emotions and reduces the need for worry to take away the negative emotions. • Assists clients in reducing use of avoidance and safety behaviors.
Acceptance	• Helps clients accept that there will always be some amount of uncertainty no matter what they do to try to rid themselves of it. • Helps clients see that the process of trying to get rid of the uncertainty can actually trigger negative emotions.

3.3　Factors that Influence Treatment Decisions

3.3.1　Age, Sex, and Ethnicity

CBT has been found to be useful for children, adolescents, and adults of all ages. In younger children, age-appropriate strategies may need to be employed. CBT appears to be equally effective for males and females with GAD. Cultural issues should be considered in treating people with GAD. Although little research has been conducted on adapting the treatment for different cultural groups, therapists should pay special attention to whether some worries are considered normal for that particular culture (e.g., "if I didn't worry about my kids, I would be a bad mother"). Furthermore, CBT is often directive, and some clients of different cultures may not respond as well to this type of treatment.

3.3.2　Education

CBT is appropriate for individuals from a wide range of educational backgrounds. In working with clients from lower education levels, assessment, homework, and therapeutic strategies may need to be adjusted. That is, these areas may need to be simplified so that the client can understand and participate fully.

3.3.3   Family and Relationship Factors

Including family members in therapy can be important for the treatment. If the family member is supportive, he or she can be a valuable asset in helping the client achieve his or her goals. However, interpersonal difficulties with family members may lead to barriers in treatment. Thus, it is a good idea to fully assess the closeness of these family relationships and how these relationships interact with the client's symptoms.

3.3.4   Client Preference

It is important for the client to participate in deciding on goals of treatment and treatment plans because giving the client this responsibility has been shown to improve outcome of treatment. It is useful to help the client come up with treatment goals and to help guide the process as much as possible. It is also important to have the client describe his or her expectations and to let the client know to what degree those expectations seem reasonable based on likely treatment outcome. That said, it is important to provide the client with hope by assuring him or her that the treatment has been effective in many research studies.

3.3.5   Treatment History

Assessment of treatment history is important when making treatment recommendations. If the client has undergone treatment previously, it is important to find out what has worked and what has not worked in that previous treatment. This assessment can help with anticipating potential obstacles and dealing with those potential obstacles. Furthermore, current therapy can often build on strategies that have worked in the past.

3.3.6   Ability to Articulate Cognitions

Because much of the experience of GAD is related to worry, it is important that the client can articulate his or her worries and the cognitions related to worry. Most components of treatment (i.e., cognitive therapy, worry exposure, and acceptance strategies) will depend on the ability of the client to articulate the nature of his or her worries.

3.3.7   Severity of Positive Beliefs About Worry

The degree to which the person believes that worry is helpful is important to learn before therapy begins. If worry is "ego-syntonic" (i.e., the person views his or her worry as an important part of his or her identity), it could prove to be a barrier to reducing worry. That is, some clients will see their worry as reducing the likelihood of a bad event or as highly adaptive. If the client views worry in this way, then he or she may be motivated to continue worrying and thus may be resistant to working on the worry. Furthermore, a person might present with wanting to work on the muscle tension and may not see worry as the cause of this muscle tension (e.g., he or she actually may see the worry as a coping mechanism).

3.3.8　Comorbidities

If a person presents with multiple psychological problems, it is useful to determine which of these manifold problems is the most important to change (i.e., the primary problem). The primary problem is usually the one that causes the most significant impairment and distress. Asking the client to identify the problem he or she would most like to fix often leads to a description of the primary problem. It is important for the therapist and client to discuss how comorbid problems affect the client and whether these problems will constitute a barrier in treatment. Although multiple problems can be worked on simultaneously (e.g., minor depression with GAD), more severe comorbid problems may warrant psychological treatment before working on GAD.

4

Treatment

4.1   Methods of CBT

Treatment of GAD typically lasts between 10 and 15 weekly sessions. Sessions usually last between 50 min and an hour, but exposure-based sessions may last somewhat longer, frequently between 90 min and 2 hr. Therapy often includes a variety of strategies, including psychoeducation procedures, cognitive strategies, exposure-based strategies, relaxation and acceptance strategies, as well as methods to reduce or prevent relapse. This section discusses each of these strategies in detail.

This structure is quite flexible in that clients will be able to progress through therapy topics at a different pace. Thus, this structure can be seen as a recipe, which will be modified based on the "tastes" of the client. At times, the client may not fully understand or be able to fully implement the techniques associated with a particular approach. We like to think that even though the client has not fully grasped the concept involved, a seed has been planted that may germinate in time. That is, the client may not fully understand how to implement the technique in practice until time has passed. Additionally, the structure presented herein is specified for a person with only a diagnosis of GAD. For people with comorbid disorders, additional time might need to be spent on specific topics. Finally, other events can occur in a person's life that might take away attention from the following structure. Hence, this structure is seen as a rough sketch of a therapy structure for someone with GAD. The boxes below provide an example of a session-by-session summary of topics covered in a 10-session therapy.

Session 1

- Develop agenda in collaboration with client
- Discuss assessment and diagnosis
- Discuss and develop initial case conceptualization in collaboration with client
- Introduce GAD treatment strategies
- Assign homework of reading over case conceptualization

Overall, the goal of this session is to plan the course of therapy with the client. We find that it is very important to provide the client with a great deal of hope in this session. That is, it is important to raise the client's expectancies that this therapy is designed for him or her and has been quite successful in previous clients and in research studies. It is also important to have the client take responsibility for change. Having the client participate in conceptualization and treatment planning can help him or her feel responsible for change and enhance his or her sense of self-efficacy. As mentioned above, clients may not fully understand everything that is discussed immediately. Thus, it is important to let them know that some topics might not instantly lead to change and that it takes time for those ideas to germinate before they are fully formed.

Session 2

- Develop agenda in collaboration with client
- Review of homework and cognitive model of GAD
- Discuss intolerance of uncertainty model and how it influences client's worry
- Identify manifestations of intolerance of uncertainty
- Assign homework of monitoring worry and situations with need for certainty

The focus of this session is explaining the model of intolerance of uncertainty. This topic can be difficult sometimes for clients to understand. Bringing in examples from the client's life can be helpful. The therapist should explain that no one loves uncertainty, and it is normal to want to know what is going to happen. However, this need to know, in the extreme, leads to problems. It is important to emphasize that much of what the client does is normal, but that doing too much of it (e.g., excessive worry) leads to problems (distress).

Session 3

- Develop agenda in collaboration with client
- Review of homework and intolerance of uncertainty model
- Discuss positive beliefs about worry model
- Identify and evaluate positive beliefs about worry
- Assign homework of pros and cons of worry

A review of the intolerance of uncertainty model is very important in this session. We encourage the client to bring up instances in the past week when he or she noticed intolerance of uncertainty. Investigating what happened during those situations is vital. The new topic for this session is positive beliefs about worry. That is, the client is asked to identify how worry is beneficial. The WWS-II and the COWS can be helpful to generate positive beliefs about worry. As mentioned above, worry is part of normal adaptive functioning. However, for a person with GAD, worry has diminishing returns (and harmful effects).

In this session, multiple topics are investigated. Reviewing positive beliefs about worry and intolerance of uncertainty is important. Furthermore, new topics such as metaworry, overestimates of the probability of risk, and catastrophizing are discussed. We find that keeping old newspaper clippings of headlines describing doomsday scenarios are helpful in illustrating the idea that all of us are prone to worry. Although the headlines may have led to a great deal of

Session 4

- Develop agenda in collaboration with client
- Review of homework, positive beliefs about worry, and intolerance of uncertainty
- Describe metaworry model
- Assess usefulness of worrying about worry
- Discuss interpretation bias of ambiguous stimuli
- Evaluate probability and risk in assessment of ambiguous stimuli
- Discuss tendency to catastrophize feared outcomes and its consequences
- Assign cognitive homework of evaluating risk

anxiety, the worst possible scenario rarely happened. This process can parallel the client's worries. That is, discussing instances of past worries and how the feared situation actually turned out can show the client that the worst is often expected, but rarely occurs.

Session 5

- Develop agenda in collaboration with client
- Review of homework
- Describe worry as cognitive avoidance strategy
- Discuss how worry as a cognitive avoidance strategy fits in with previous models
- Describe rationale for worry exposure
- Assign homework

This session is vital in setting up the rationale for exposure-based techniques. If the client can understand how he or she jumps from worry to worry, then he or she will be more likely to understand why exposure is important.

Session 6

- Develop agenda in collaboration with client
- Review of homework and rationale for worry exposure
- Conduct worry exposure
- Assign homework of worry exposure

This session is the first session in which worry exposure occurs. It is important to stay with the worry and not let the person jump to another worry (this is admittedly easier said than done). For a beginning therapist, exposures can be very difficult emotionally, and the emotions involved will make both the client and therapist uncomfortable. It is very tempting to help the client minimize those emotions. However, it is vital to the client that the therapist stays calm and keeps the client in the exposure. The homework that is assigned should be very similar to the exposure done in session. The goal of homework is to practice skills that are learned in therapy. It is unwise to give the person homework that was not practiced in session. As part of this therapy structure, this session could be repeated to allow for another opportunity for the client to practice the worry exposure with the therapist. It is critical for the client to learn that he or she can handle the emotions that go with sticking with a worry. The client may also learn the important message that he or she can cope much better than imagined.

Session 7

- Develop agenda in collaboration with client
- Review of homework and more worry exposure if needed
- Discuss intolerance of uncertainty in terms of acceptance
- Assign homework of acceptance of uncertainty

This session has similar components to an earlier session that described intolerance of uncertainty. However, it adds in a component of acceptance. That is, the therapist and client will have a discussion about how the client might be less anxious and worried if he or she practiced acceptance.

Session 8

- Develop agenda in collaboration with client
- Review of homework and acceptance of uncertainty
- Assign homework of more acceptance of uncertainty

The last three sessions of therapy focus on reviewing previous skills, addressing deficits of skills, and providing the client with a great deal of positive reinforcement of the skills that he or she has developed. A potent message that should be provided to the client is that he or she has the skills to handle his or her worry in a more productive manner – that is, to really develop autonomy.

Session 9

- Develop agenda in collaboration with client
- Review of homework
- Review treatment gains in terms of original case conceptualization
- Assign homework of most effective strategies learned in therapy

---

This session is designed to assist the client with relapse prevention, and it will be important to review the skills and concepts that help the client reduce his or her worry. It is also important to discuss difficult situations in the future that might cause his or her worry to return or be exacerbated. It is important to plan for difficulties in the future and to indicate to the client that he or she can handle those difficulties.

Session 10

- Develop agenda in collaboration with client
- Discuss homework and treatment gains
- Discuss goals for the future that the client would like to continue
- Discuss potential barriers that might lead to "slips" in excessive worry

This session is similar to session 9 in that relapse prevention is emphasized. This session can be used to discuss what the client will do as he or she takes over the role of "therapist."

4.1.1   Psychoeducation

In the psychoeducation sessions of treatment, the therapist provides the client with information about the outcome of the assessment (i.e., diagnosis and case conceptualization), different models of worry, and the basics of CBT. It is also important to instill a hopeful attitude in the client. That is, the client is most likely to succeed when he or she has high expectancies for therapy.

Assessment Outcome and Case Conceptualization
It can be very helpful for the client to understand the assessment process, what each of the measures assessed, and how the assessment guides the diagnosis and treatment planning. In the past, clients may have been explicitly told they have the diagnosis of GAD, but they may not understand completely what this diagnosis means. It is important to explain that GAD is a disorder in which the person has excessive and uncontrollable worry. Worry can be explained as a natural tendency that everyone has. However, to qualify for the diagnosis, the worry must be excessive and cause functional impairment in the person's life. That is, worry is a normal phenomenon, but the client's worry has become enough of a problem that an intervention is needed to bring it back in line with normal functioning. A potential analogy is to discuss diabetes and how the goal of diabetes treatment is to bring the person's level of glucose to a manageable level. Similarly, the goal of treatment is to bring worry down to a more manageable level where it does not impair functioning. However, it is important to note to the client that eliminating worry is not a goal of treatment.

It is also helpful to discuss the client's case conceptualization with him or her (an excellent resource for case conceptualization of anxiety disorders is Butler, Fennell, & Hackmann, 2008). A case conceptualization helps someone make sense of his or her problems by fitting the person's problems into accepted models. The conceptualization creates a map of how the person arrived at his or her current level of functioning. It also provides a diagram of the process of worry and identifies situations in which the maladaptive patterns can be broken so the person can function at a better level.

The treatment of diabetes can be a useful metaphor for understanding the treatment of GAD

An important part of the therapeutic process is to have the client "buy into" the model being used. Having him or her become a part of the "blueprint" of his or her treatment can assist in this process of buying into therapy. Furthermore, it also is expected that the client will act as his or her own therapist following treatment. Thus, it is helpful to have the client be very aware of the causes of his or her problems and what strategies will be implemented in therapy to break the links in this excessive worry process.

Case conceptualization should be created and discussed with the client

Diagrams and metaphors can be very useful in helping the client understand the conceptualization being used. Sample diagrams will be provided throughout the following sections, in the sample case review, and in the Appendix. Figure 7, in Chapter 5, displays a case conceptualization for Laura, who is described in the clinical case vignette in that chapter. This diagram should be shown to the client. Having the client provide feedback on the conceptualization can give the client a sense of control of, and enhance the client's sense of responsibility for, what occurs during therapy. A blank conceptualization is provided in the Appendix.

Models of Worry

It is important to have the client involved in understanding how his or her excessive worry manifested. Thus, it is also important to discuss the different models of worry to see how these models fit into his or her pattern of worrying. If a client feels that the model fits his or her worry process, then the client will be more likely to buy into the treatment for breaking this process. Each of the treatments for the five models of worry (information processing, function of worry, metaworry, intolerance of uncertainty, and cognitive avoidance) will be discussed in the following sections.

Format of Cognitive Behavioral Therapy

There are certain principles of CBT that are important to describe to the client. Taking the time to identify the objectives of each phase of treatment and to describe fully what will happen in therapy will reduce the likelihood that the client will be surprised later in treatment. Similarly, clients who are asked for feedback on the treatment process (e.g., "What was this experience like?"

CBT Treatment of GAD: Principles to Discuss with Client

The goal is to equip clients with the tools necessary to allow them to deal with their problems independently

A main goal of this treatment is to provide clients with the knowledge and skills to deal with their excessive worry independently. It is the clients' responsibility to practice and learn new skills. Only hard work will reduce the client's excessive worry. The therapist is responsible for teaching skills in an accessible manner and providing motivation (i.e., helping to expose clients' intrinsic motivation) and hope to the clients. The therapist does not have a secret formulation of therapy. All formulations and plans are shared with clients, and the clients are responsible for providing feedback on the development of the formulation.

CBT is present-focused

Although some description of the etiological factors responsible for the development of the excessive worry may be helpful to the client, the focus of therapy is on what is currently maintaining the problem and what will be helpful to reducing it. CBT is a pragmatic and present-centered therapy.

Treatment is directive and short-term

Because a goal of CBT is to help clients become their own therapists, treatment is short-term. Because of the limited amount of time available, a great deal of planning and hard work will be necessary to prepare the client for independence. Thus, the client needs to focus on the treatment strategies to reduce their worry. If the client is reluctant to make the change, then this type of therapy might not be suitable until the client is ready. Moreover, the client must be ready to engage in the sometimes difficult work involved in reducing their worry. However, if engagement occurs, the difficulty is relatively short-lived, and gains can be expected.

"What did you find helpful?") may benefit by feeling fully involved and responsible for their treatment success. Some of the most important aspects of CBT that should be discussed with the client are described below.

4.1.2   Cognitive Strategies

A number of cognitive strategies will be employed to break the cycle of worry in the client. These strategies fit well with previously discussed models of GAD (see Chapter 2). Specifically, the cognitive strategies will dovetail with the following models of worry: intolerance of uncertainty, positive beliefs about worry, metaworry, and information-processing biases.

It is important for the therapist and client to discuss the relationship between intolerance of uncertainty and excessive worry

Intolerance of Uncertainty and Excessive Worry

The first step is to describe and point out the links between intolerance of uncertainty and worry. That is, if the person could tolerate more uncertainty, then he or she would not need to worry excessively. It should be shown that worry is a strategy for reducing uncertainty. Specifically, worry typically extends to all potential situations, and this excessive mental activity is a cognitive strategy used to reduce uncertainty.

A second step in this cognitive strategy is to discuss whether certainty can ever be attained, having the client explore how achievable the goal of absolute certainty is. As the client decides that certainty is not a possibility, motivational interviewing techniques can be used to weigh the costs of trying to attain certainty against the benefits of tolerating more uncertainty. Said another way, the client can weigh the pros and cons of trying to attain certainty.

A third step in the cognitive strategy is to observe and detail when this need for certainty arises and how the client uses worry to reduce this need. Specifically, it is important to monitor the antecedents and consequences of when the need for certainty arises. The therapist should give the client a monitoring form to help him or her identify these situations. It will be important to spend time in therapy going over explicitly how to fill out these forms (see the Appendix for an example). It is quite likely that the client is not even aware of how trying to reduce the need for certainty leads to automatic thoughts (e.g., something bad will happen) and behaviors (e.g., calling one's daughter repeatedly). Other examples of these behaviors include (1) seeking reassurance from others before making a decision or obtaining excessive information about a topic, and (2) procrastinating on making a decision until the deadline approaches so that the negative emotions associated with being uncertain are time limited.

A fourth step in this cognitive strategy is to experience situations that induce uncertainty and to develop strategies for coping in these situations. The goal of this step is to have clients experience the anxiety associated with uncertainty but to see that they can deal with the anxiety without relying on a mental strategy to reduce uncertainty. This type of skill training is similar to what occurs during the exposure therapy sessions (described below). Furthermore, the acceptance-based strategies will also be helpful in dealing with uncertainty (described more below).

Positive Beliefs of Worry

Another cognitive strategy is to focus on how positive beliefs about worry interact with intolerance of uncertainty to reinforce worry. That is, the client may see worry as being beneficial and may be ambivalent about change because of these perceived positive benefits. If this is the case, it is often useful to explore with the client all of the positive benefits of worry, with the therapist acting in an open and accepting manner (i.e., the therapist must be willing to listen to all explanations in a nonjudgmental manner). Most likely, worry has actually helped the client in some situations in the past. Next, the client and therapist can discuss any potential negative outcomes that result from worry. Then, a particular focus may be directed to the long-term problems with worry and how the worry can reinforce itself. By discussing the pros and cons of worry in this motivational interviewing style, the therapist can permit the client to decide on whether worry is beneficial. Furthermore, if the client makes the decision that there are downsides to worry, then he or she is also likely to take the responsibility for the goal to reduce worry. It is likely that clients will be more invested in reducing worry if they are the ones to formulate reasons their worry is not beneficial. The endorsed items on the WW-II (Freeston et al., 1994) and the COWS (Davey et al., 1996) are both good places to start the discussion of positive beliefs about worry.

Metaworry

It is important to discuss how metaworry, or worry about worry, can actually lead to more anxiety. That is, clients can be encouraged to discuss how their worry about worrying actually leads them to feel more anxiety and possibly to worry more. Once the client sees this pattern, the costs and benefits of worry about worry should be discussed in a similar manner as was suggested above for positive beliefs in worry. The person might decide that when a "worry about worry" thought arrives it is best to just ignore it. Additionally, the acceptance-based practice of noticing a thought and letting it go (explained below) can also be useful in dampening the influence of metaworry.

Cognitive Biases

Because individuals with GAD exhibit interpretation and attention biases in the direction of threat, it will be important to address these biases in treatment. With regards to interpretation biases (see Chapter 2), therapy will need to address the individual's tendency to overestimate the likelihood of the feared outcome (biased probability estimates) as well as the tendency to assume that the worst will happen (catastrophizing). Labeling thoughts as distortions opens up the possibility that other alternative thoughts can exist, and it helps the client to experience some emotional distance from the thought (and thus develop more control over the worry). Additionally, once these biases are exposed, clients can challenge them and create more realistic assessments of the situations that had induced worry. It is important to point out to the client that the act of challenging thoughts does not consist of substituting positive thoughts for negative thoughts. More accurately, the goal of cognitive therapy is to examine all the evidence, and in the case of GAD, to recognize that events occur less often and with less catastrophic outcomes than expected.

Specific to overestimating the probability of an event occurring, several challenging questions can be used by the therapist and then taught to the client. For example, it is helpful to have the client give a percentage estimate for the event occurring (e.g., "On a scale of 0 to 100%, how sure are you that your worry will come true?"). Once the overestimate is labeled (e.g., "90%"), the therapist and client can challenge this estimate. For example, a therapist can reframe this estimate by pointing out that this estimate assumes that the feared outcome occurs 9 out of 10 times. Usually, this reframe illuminates that fact that the estimate was way too high, and a more realistic estimate can then be discussed. Another useful tool for challenging overestimates of risk is to have the client start to record how often worries actually come true. If clients are in fact overestimating the likelihood of an event, then there will be many times when a feared outcome does not come true. This record can be used to dispute this interpretation bias.

In the case of catastrophizing, the therapist and client can explore the client's tendency to engage in this distortion. Next, the therapist and client can challenge the catastrophic thought by exploring possible alternative outcomes to the feared one. Clients should be encouraged to generate these alternative outcomes whenever they notice that they are catastrophizing. Occasionally, a client feels completely sure that the feared outcome is likely. In this case, helping the client to "worry though" the fear (i.e., explore the consequences by asking questions like "So what?" or "Then what happens?") can help the client to see that he or she can survive the worst possible outcome.

Common to most CBT are records of situations, thoughts, emotions, and behaviors. Similar to the monitoring suggested for intolerance of uncertainty, it may be helpful for the client to monitor their worry with "worry records" (e.g., Craske & Barlow, 2006). Worry records force the client to detail the characteristics of a worry (e.g., the duration of the worry, the level of anxiety and types of physical symptoms experienced during the worry, the triggering event, and the thoughts and behaviors associated with the worry). Interpretation biases and probability assumptions can also be addressed with the worry record by adding in sections for "alternative possibilities" and "real odds" (Craske & Barlow, 2006). The continued practice of generating possible alternatives and assessing risk appropriately helps the client see that the feared outcome is not necessarily the most likely outcome.

> **Self-monitoring of worry often helps clients identify and challenge distorted thinking**

Because individuals with GAD also demonstrate an attention bias towards threatening material, which may have direct effects on worry, clients should also be taught to attend to positive outcomes (Roemer & Orsillo, 2002). The therapist can point out that the client may only be attending to negative and threatening aspects of their environment and that this attention bias increases their tendency to worry. Clients should be encouraged to start documenting positive outcomes to events so that they can learn to direct their attention away from threat.

4.1.3   Exposure-Based Strategies

The goal of exposure in GAD is to help the person see the worry as a cognitive avoidance strategy and to experience the negative emotion without using worry to avoid it. Prior to conducting exposure, the model for intolerance of uncertainty should be reviewed. A discussion of how intolerance of uncertainty leads to negative emotions and how worry is used as a way of dealing with the negative emotions is important in explaining the reasons for exposure.

Taking an aspirin is an example of negative reinforcement that may be a helpful metaphor in therapy

After reviewing intolerance of uncertainty, the client and therapist should discuss how worry is negatively reinforced. It may be useful to describe negative reinforcement using the example of taking an aspirin. Aspirin is a tool that people use when they want to do something about their negative sensations. Likewise, worry is a tool that people use to reduce or avoid negative emotions. That is, worry only provides a superficial examination of the person's concerns. Because these tools are effective in diminishing negative states, their use to diminish future negative states is reinforced (i.e., negative reinforcement). Worry is effective as a negative reinforcer because by worrying in words rather than in mental images, the person avoids some of the negative emotions he or she would have felt if they had fully processed the situation. However, a problem exists with this strategy: Avoiding images does not allow the person to experience the natural reduction of negative emotions that would occur after processing them for a few minutes.

It might be helpful for the therapist to illustrate the process of exposure in reducing fear by reference to specific phobias. For example, the therapist might describe how a person who fears elevators could choose to take the stairs to avoid the elevator. But by taking the stairs, he does not experience the fear of the elevator and, thereby, fails to see how the fear reduces naturally over time. The worry in GAD is analogous to taking the stairs. In particular, the person never thinks through the issue completely, thus never realizing that he or she will usually have the ability to cope. Consequently, the worry maintains perceptions of high danger levels. Similarly, the person taking the stairs instead of the elevator feels reduced anxiety because he avoided the "dangerous" elevator. Therefore, the person continues to believe that the elevator is dangerous. Additionally, they never experience the counterevidence that would prove that the elevator is not dangerous. Similarly, a person jumping from worry to worry never learns that he or she can cope with the negative emotions associated with one specific worry.

The exposures for the cognitive avoidance aspect of GAD include two elements: (1) the mental image of the threatening stimuli, and (2) the negative emotions associated with this image. The image should be related to a worry that the person often has. For example, the person might frequently worry about his or her work situation (see Table 6). An exposure for this worry could have the client process and focus on what it would mean to lose his job. The person would imagine all the details of losing his job as vividly as possible and feel the negative emotions associated with this imagery (e.g., what he would do the first day after losing his job, from the first thing in the morning until the end of the day).

It is important for clients to keep focused on the image being used in exposure therapy

As mentioned before, people with GAD will jump from worry to worry so as not to fully experience the negative emotions. In the exposure, it is important to keep them focused on the image that has been selected and not let them start jumping to other worries. In the example above, the person might try to jump from the image of losing the job to other worries, such as paying medical bills or addressing health concerns. It is important to keep the client focused

Table 6
Example of Exposure to a Client's Worry and the Downward Arrow Technique

"I might lose my job"

↓

Therapist: "What would happen if you lost your job"

↓

"I would not be able to afford things"

↓

Therapist: "What types of things might you not be able to afford"

↓

"I would not be able to afford food or clothes"

↓

Therapist: "So you would have no job and not be able to buy food or clothes"

↓

"Yeah, and I would have nothing to do but watch TV"

↓

Therapist: "Let's focus on that image. You are home with nothing to do, watching TV in your pajamas, with nothing to eat."

on the content of one worry (losing his job) and how the worried outcome will affect the client. The downward arrow technique can be helpful in finding the core of the worry. The therapist can ask questions such as:

"What might happen next?"

"What could that lead to?"

"What would be so bad about that?"

The goal of exposures is to have the person keep the imagery in focus and to experience the associated negative emotion. Quite often, clients will get to a point where they see that they would be able to cope with the situation. For example, they are likely to report, "I guess I would start looking for a job" or "I am sure I would have some food because I am getting unemployment benefits."

If the client is also avoiding situations or using subtle avoidance behaviors (e.g., reassurance seeking), an additional session may be needed to address these behaviors with exposure techniques. The therapist and client should brainstorm all the avoidant and safety behaviors that the client engages in, detailing those situations that would be more or less difficult (i.e., anxiety provoking). Then the situations can be ranked, and the client and therapist can jointly create a fear-and-avoidance hierarchy. For homework the client can start to face the feared and avoided situations during the time between sessions. The client's goal should be to work through all of the items on the hierarchy. It is important that each item be faced repeatedly so that the client can habituate to the anxiety that the situations provoke.

It is also important for the therapist to help motivate the client to engage in certain challenging behaviors and situations (an entire session can be spent on motivation enhancement if necessary). The therapist can enhance the client's motivation by helping the client to see that the time spent on worry, avoidance, and safety will conflict and interfere with other valued actions. One way to highlight this discrepancy is to have the client list all of the areas in his or her life that are important. One can identify an area's value by using the amount of time spent on an area as an indicator of its importance. Using time as an indicator is helpful because of time's limited nature, and because there are finite constraints on how much time we can spend on each valued area. The therapist can suggest that although worry may not be seen as valuable, the client is currently spending a lot of time engaged in worry. The valued areas can be drawn into a pie diagram based on how much time is given to each (an example is provided in the Appendix; adapted from Fairburn, 2008). For an individual with GAD, the pie chart can demonstrate that worry consumes a predominant slice of the pie, which necessarily reduces the amount of time the client can spend on other important areas. The therapist and client can brainstorm ways to reduce the worry piece while also considering how to increase the other valued pieces. The therapist can point out that the techniques used in treatment, such as exposure, can help (1) to reduce worry and (2) to increase valued time in those areas of life for which the exposure is relevant.

4.1.4   Relaxation and Acceptance-Based Strategies

Acceptance-based strategies target experiential avoidance (i.e., situations in which one attempts to alter the intensity or frequency of unwanted negative internal experiences; Hayes, Wilson, Gifford, Follette, & Strosahl, 1996). People with GAD use worry as a means of escaping or avoiding negative emotional experiences. Engaging in the worry process reduces physiological reactivity and distracts worriers from more distressing topics. Directly targeting how individuals respond to internal experiences may enhance the treatment of GAD.

Efforts to avoid internal experiences paradoxically worsen distress

The first part of this strategy is to highlight the client's habitual nature of anxious responding (i.e., the automatic way that the client responds). Additionally, the therapist and client can discuss how efforts to avoid internal experiences paradoxically worsen distress. The client explores and learns to change his or her relationship to internal experience. The goal is for the client to become more aware and more able to use emotional responses as information. This information can act as a guide, and the awareness allows the client to choose whether or not to go where these emotions lead.

Clients are taught a variety of mindfulness practices, many of which are drawn from Kabat-Zinn (1994; Kabat-Zinn et al., 1992) and Segal, Williams, & Teasdale (2001). Mindfulness refers to awareness of the present moment, a condition in which the thoughts, emotions, and sensations of the present are acknowledged and accepted. The objectives of mindfulness practices are to enhance the client's ability to stay focused in the present moment and to encourage the client to experience all emotions, thoughts, and sensation without judgment (i.e., to get the client to see these experiences as a natural and necessary part of the present moment). Clients can be taught the practice of "noticing and letting go." For example, when the client feels distress, he or she can note the distress and then observe how the distress dissipates. Clients are encouraged to practice mindfulness both in planned exercises and while engaging in typical activities. These activities help the client become aware of emotional states. Then, the client can make decisions on whether to engage in his or her habitual behavior (i.e., engaging in worry) or to accept the negative emotion and move forward.

It is useful to have clients learn to pay attention to bodily sensations. For example, people with GAD often have high amounts of muscular tension. The first step in mindfulness training might be to pay attention to the muscular tension throughout the day (a tracking sheet can be created if that assists the client). As the person becomes more aware of bodily sensations, he or she might become more aware of the emotional reactions that preceded that tension, and he or she will notice the transient nature of these states. That is, a person is likely to experience a strong emotional reaction that dissipates as time passes.

> **Mindfulness techniques promote an understanding of the transient nature of emotional and physical states**

If desired or necessary, an additional session can be used for relaxation training, depending on the interest of the client. The therapist can guide a client through progressive muscle relaxation (PMR), or both therapist and client can listen to a prerecorded relaxation tape. A copy of the recording can be given to the client for continued practice. PMR fits well with mindfulness practices because it asks participants to practice noticing thoughts and letting them go. It is important to explain to the client that these exercises should not be used to avoid anxiety but to practice being mindful. Free scripts for PMR can be found online (e.g., http://www.innerhealthstudio.com/progressive-muscle-relaxation-exercise.html).

4.2   Mechanisms of Action

4.2.1   Cognitive Models

Cognitive models of GAD assume that excessive worry comes from intolerance of uncertainty, positive beliefs about worry, and information-processing biases. That is, people with GAD feel that worry is a beneficial strategy, they interpret ambiguous events as threatening, and they cannot tolerate uncertainty (and thus they experience negative emotions when situations are uncertain; e.g., Dugas, Buhr, & Ladouceur, 2005; Dugas, Gosselin, & Ladouceur, 2001).

The intolerance of uncertainty construct has been shown to be strongly related to GAD and is thought to be a susceptibility factor for developing GAD. In fact, evidence shows that decreasing intolerance of uncertainty is an effective treatment strategy for individuals with GAD (58% of patients met high end state functioning at 12-month follow-up when treatment directly addressed intolerance of uncertainty; Ladouceur et al, 2000). Additionally, treatment that focuses on this characteristic outperformed wait list control, for both individual (e.g., Dugas and Robichaud, 2007) and group (Dugas et al., 2003) formats, and applied relaxation (Dugas & Robichaud, 2007). Moreover, Dugas and Ladouceur (2000) found that when analyzing the changes that occur during treatment, changes in intolerance of uncertainty preceded changes in worry, whereas the reverse relationship did not occur. These results indicate that cognitive change with respect to intolerance of uncertainty is important for treatment success.

With regard to positive beliefs about worry, Purdon (2000) found that positive beliefs about worry were a predictor of reduced motivation to get rid of worry. Additionally, when worry is reinforced by the various mechanisms described earlier (e.g., cognitive avoidance, negative reinforcement), the positive beliefs about worry are also reinforced. Treatments that take into account the effect of positive beliefs about worry on the maintenance of worry have been found to successfully reduce worry and anxiety (e.g., 75% of individuals met criteria for recovery at 12-month follow-up; Wells & King, 2006).

Emerging evidence shows the importance of attention re-training for individuals with GAD

There is consistent evidence that individuals with GAD evince an attentional bias to threatening environmental cues (Mogg & Bradley, 2005) and tend to interpret ambiguous stimuli as threatening (Eysenck et al., 1987; Eysenck et al., 1991; Mathews et al., 1989; Mogg et al., 1994). These biases suggest that addressing these cognitive propensities in treatment is important. With respect to interpretation biases, there is evidence that one can help individuals with GAD to access less threatening interpretations and that these interpretations lead to less worry intrusions (Hayes, Hirsch, Krebs, & Mathews, 2010). With respect to attention biases, treatments that retrain individuals to attend to less threatening stimuli (with simple computer tasks) lead to a decrease in the biased attention to threat. The effect sizes of this attention retraining task are similar to those found for CBT (50% of treated individuals were classified as responders; Amir, Beard, Burns, & Bomyea, 2009). Similarly, another study found that using a computerized task to train individuals not to engage with threat meanings led those individuals to worry less (Hirsch et al., 2010). Although the treatment purported in this book does not make use of computerized attention training, teaching clients to become aware of positive and nonthreatening elements in their daily environments may have similar effects.

In sum, cognitive strategies are thought to work on the components mentioned above by (1) assessing the usefulness of worry as a strategy in light of the difficulties associated with it, (2) assisting in reframing ambiguous situations in a more realistic light rather than as threatening, and (3) helping the client investigate whether the pursuit of certainty is useful or even possible. Said differently, cognitive strategies shift thinking patterns by examining the evidence and replacing worry-provoking thoughts with more realistic and balanced beliefs.

4.2.2   Behavioral and Emotional Processing Models

Although cognitive strategies are beneficial in the ways mentioned above, successful treatment of GAD requires use of experiential techniques, such as exposure. In Chapter 2, worry was discussed as a cognitive avoidance strategy, which allowed the person to escape deeply processing negative stimuli. This avoidance of experience must be challenged so that individuals can learn that the stimuli they fear are not necessarily harmful. Once this successful learning takes place, the reinforcement of worry can be dampened. Another reason more experiential methods such as exposures are necessary is because cognitive strategies may be verbally rule governed. As we saw earlier, verbally rule-governed strategies may preclude an individual from experiencing competing (and in this case, contradictory) environmental information. The use of exposures (focusing on images rather than words) without distraction (without using the verbal process of worry) can allow the competing environmental information to be processed, thus allowing the individual to learn that the feared images are not inherently dangerous.

Exposure strategies are used so that the person can fully process the stimuli nonverbally. Exposure therapy is considered the first line of treatment for many anxiety disorders because of its success in reducing fear and avoidance. It is thought that exposure techniques work through a number of mechanisms including extinction learning (Myers & Davis, 2007; Quirk & Mueller, 2008;) and changing the fear network (Foa & Kozak, 1986; through fully processing the emotional information). In the case of exposure to fearful stimuli, extinction works by reducing anxiety through repeatedly presenting the situation without the expected punishment. A person who engages in exposure would see that the negative emotion is not as bad as expected. This process is thought to be active in that the person is learning new information to take the place of previous information. Thus, the person learns that he or she can handle negative emotions and that he or she is able to cope without having to escape from the situation.

It is also thought that extinction strategies assist the person in rewriting the fear that is associated in memory. Foa and Kozak (1986) maintain that we store fear memories in a fear network. This network is accessed as the person is exposed to the threatening stimulus. The information in the network is rewritten as the person is exposed to the negative stimuli without negative consequences. Thus, the person is able to react differently to the stimuli that led them to worry.

Because successful exposure therapy requires the feared stimuli to be present, exposure therapy with GAD can be tricky. This difficulty exists because the range of feared stimuli in GAD is broad rather than specific as in other anxiety disorders. It will be important for the client to think of many different types of worries so that the treatment can be effective. Additionally, although most of the focus in treatment is placed on cognitive avoidance (avoiding fearful images), the mechanisms explained above apply to any behavioral avoidance in which the individual engages. Thus, exposure to those avoided situations will also reduce avoidance and fear of those situations in the manner mentioned above.

4.2.3   Acceptance-Based Models

Acceptance-based treatment techniques attempt to reduce the avoidance of negative emotions, by experiencing and accepting these emotions without judgment

Hayes and colleagues (Hayes et al., 1996; 1999) have proposed that anxiety and other difficulties come from our attempt to control or diminish internal experience. People with GAD attempt to avoid negative thoughts and feelings (see Roemer & Orsillo, 2002), but these attempts are unsuccessful and have paradoxical effects. Additionally, the use of worry, which is verbal, prevents awareness of internal and external experiences. Although exposure-based treatments are largely experiential, acceptance and mindfulness can be used to directly access and process experiences. A person who notices and accepts the negative emotions without trying to do something to reduce the emotions will see the negative emotion disappear (similar to what occurs in exposure). If a person attempts to avoid an emotion, this person will paradoxically increase these negative events (emotions) in the long run. Similarly, focusing on avoiding thoughts and feelings prevents an individual from engaging with the environment in a meaningful way. Specifically, the aforementioned strategy may prevent the individual from spending time doing something the individual values. Additionally, avoidance keeps individuals from spending time trying to change aspects of the environment that are troubling. Indeed, Sarah Hayes, Susan Orsillo, and Lizabeth Roemer (Hayes, Orsillo, & Roemer, 2010) found that increasing one's acceptance of internal experience produced a significantly greater response to treatment and a higher self-reported quality of life for individuals with GAD.

4.3   Efficacy and Prognosis

4.3.1   Efficacy of CBT

This section discusses the efficacy of general CBT compared with different control conditions. Information regarding the efficacy of different types of CBT for GAD (e.g., intolerance of uncertainty, metaworry) is included in Section 4.2 where available. Reviews of treatment outcome studies (e.g., Borkovec & Ruscio, 2001; Gould, Safren, Washington, & Otto, 2004) suggest that CBT for GAD was more effective than no treatment and control treatments, with large effect sizes ranging from 0.71 to 0.90 (Galenberg et al., 2000; Moller, Volz, Reimann, & Stoll, 2001; Rickels, Pollack, Sheehan, & Haskins, 2000). Moreover, CBT reduces worry (the cardinal feature of GAD), as measured by the PSWQ, by an effect size of −1.15 (Covin, Ouimet, Seeds, & Dozois, 2008). Gains from treatment seem to be maintained over time. Clinical improvement can be seen in around 38% to 63% of clients who complete treatment (Waters & Craske, 2005). These numbers are not as high as CBT for other anxiety disorders (e.g., CBT for panic disorders results in approximately 80% of clients experiencing clinical improvement; Campbell & Brown, 2002).

Studies show that cognitive, behavioral, mindfulness, and relaxation techniques are all effective treatment strategies for GAD

Other researchers are adding components of mindfulness (e.g., increasing acceptance of internal experiences; Roemer, Orsillo, & Salters-Pedneault, 2008) to improve the effectiveness of existing treatments. Roemer and colleagues have been successful in adding the mindfulness components to existing treatments. In fact, 78% of individuals diagnosed with GAD no longer met criteria for the disorder after receiving a behavioral treatment with mindfulness components. However, there is mixed evidence as to which components of CBT make the most difference. Some studies show that more elements (cognitive restructuring, relaxation, in vivo exposure) are better than treatment with relaxation and in vivo exposure alone (Butler, Fennell, Robson, & Gelder, 1991), whereas others found that using relaxation alone or cognitive components alone produced effects as robust as those obtained when combined treatments are used (Barlow, Rapee, & Brown, 1992).

4.4 Combination Treatments

4.4.1 Medication Treatments

Benzodiazepines are short-acting medications that reduce the physiological components of anxiety. They are often given as a short-term treatment to reduce anxiety (effect sizes range from 0.42 to 0.90; Galenberg et al., 2000; Moller et al., 2001; Rickels et al., 2000). However, the benzodiazepines have addictive properties so they are often not well suited to the treatment of GAD due to its long and chronic course. Moreover, pharmacological treatments may reduce physical symptoms of anxiety rather than worry, the predominant symptom in GAD (Anderson & Palm, 2006). Selective serotonin reuptake inhibitors (SSRIs) and tricyclic antidepressants are more desirable in that they can be used long-term without the addictive potential of benzodiazepines. SSRIs are more effective than placebo in treating GAD (Waters & Craske, 2005). Some of the potential side effects of SSRI include nausea, sexual dysfunction, headache, diarrhea, and constipation.

> SSRIs and tricyclics are more appropriate than benzodiazepines for the treatment of GAD because benzodiazepines often lead to dependency

4.4.2 Comparing and Combining Medications and CBT

Very few studies have compared the effectiveness of CBT with medication treatments for GAD. In one study (Power et al., 1990), CBT treatment (in combination with benzodiazepines or alone) displayed better outcomes (50.0–71.4% achieved clinically significant long-term change) than the benzodiazepines alone (22.3–40.9% achieved clinically significant long-term change) or the control condition (15.8–21% achieved clinically significant long-term change). Clients who received the combination treatment displayed improvement more quickly. Additionally, clients who received CBT (alone or in combination with medications) displayed the greatest long-term gains. However, more research is needed comparing the efficacy of CBT with that of medications.

> CBT in combination with medication may produce effective treatment gains

4.5 Overcoming Barriers to Treatment

This section focuses on suggestions for overcoming obstacles that occur in the context of treatment for GAD. Specific attention is given to ambivalence about treatment, homework noncompliance, and the impact of other comorbid conditions.

4.5.1 Treatment Ambivalence

People with anxiety disorders often have mixed feelings when beginning CBT treatment. It is very difficult to face fears, and generally, people experience ambivalence about changing behaviors that have somehow worked for them in the past. There are some common fears about starting CBT treatment: (1) fears that treatment will fail (e.g., "I worry this treatment won't work"), (2) fears of the consequences of the treatment succeeding (e.g., "What will happen if I don't worry?"), (3) fears that the treatment will lead to an increase in symptoms (e.g., "What happens if the treatment makes me worry more?"), (4) fears of not being able to handle the treatment (e.g., "I worry that I won't be able to go through the treatment"), and (5) miscellaneous fears (financial, treatment interfering with their work of relationships).

Motivational interviewing (Miller & Rollnick, 2002) is an approach that specifically targets treatment ambivalence. Although, much of the work on motivational interviewing has focused on substance use treatment, it is also relevant and valuable in helping people decide to make changes in other habits. Miller and Rollnick define motivational interviewing as a "client-centered, directive method for enhancing motivations to change by exploring and resolving ambivalence." The box below provides some of the key assumptions of motivational interviewing.

Key Assumptions of Motivational Interviewing

- Motivational interviewing is complementary to CBT techniques and is not an alternative to CBT.
- Clients often feel ambivalent about changing. This is a normal feeling and is not a sign of "resistance." It is not that the client is uncooperative; rather it is that the client is unsure of making changes.
- Motivation is a fluctuating state. A client may be extremely motivated for therapy at some points and very ambivalent about change at other points. Motivational interviewing does not take place only once in therapy. Motivational enhancement is continually needed throughout therapy.
- Motivational interviewing focuses on intrinsic reasons (e.g., reasons I want to change) for change more than on extrinsic reasons (e.g., reasons why they want me to change).

In motivational interviewing, the therapist is advised to take a scientific perspective that is nonjudgmental. It is important to hear both sides of the ambivalence and not make arguments for change. This process includes a thorough discussion of reasons not to change or to stay the same. A client who discovers a reason for change may be more motivated than one who is told to change. The therapist is seen as a guide for the process more than as an expert on what is important for the client. The client knows more about what is important to him or her than the therapist or other extrinsic motivators for change. The therapist "rolls with resistance" by empathetically listening and

The client who discovers a good reason for change is likely to be more motivated than one who is simply told to change

endeavoring to understand the client's ambivalence rather than arguing for change (which can paradoxically increase resistance).

A thorough discussion of motivational interviewing is beyond the scope of this book. More resources for motivational interviewing are listed in the Further Reading section of this book (Arkowitz, Westra, Miller, & Rollnick, 2008; Miller & Rollnick, 2002).

4.5.2   Homework Noncompliance

Completing homework in between sessions assists in reinforcing what has been learned in therapy. Homework is always structured so that it is a direct extension of what has been practiced in session. It helps the client continue treatment during the times when he or she is not in treatment. One means of preventing homework noncompliance is to thoroughly discuss potential barriers to completing homework after it has been assigned. This assessment may lead to the client thinking about what exactly is asked (to make sure that it is understood), identifying barriers to completing homework (e.g., time to complete it), and assessing the relevance of the assignment. However, even with a thorough discussion of potential barriers to completing homework, clients may still have difficulties completing homework.

The first step in helping the client complete his or her homework is to identify the potential reasons the homework was not completed. Some reasons for homework noncompliance include (1) the client does not feel that homework is relevant, (2) the client did not understand the homework, (3) the homework is too difficult, (4) the client has outside demands on his or her time (e.g., relationship responsibilities or busy work schedule), or (5) the therapist does not emphasize homework (e.g., does not ask about it at the next session). Once reasons for the client not completing his or her homework have been identified, the therapist can work on those specific issues.

> The therapist should help clients identify potential barriers to homework completion immediately after an assignment is given

As mentioned above, one potential way to prevent homework noncompliance is to discuss potential barriers right after the homework has been given. This practice will allow the client and therapist to brainstorm the reasons for, and barriers to, completing the homework. The therapist may also want to ask about whether the homework is too complex and whether the client will have time to complete the homework. If the client is unable to complete the homework after all of these items have been discussed, then the therapist is advised to discuss other barriers that came up that were not anticipated. In this discussion, a motivational interviewing approach of empathy and nonjudgment is likely to be helpful, and the client should be able to feel free to discuss why he or she could not complete the homework and make a decision about what can be done next time to make sure homework is completed.

Scheduling telephone contacts between sessions can also be helpful. These telephone contacts should be brief, and not duplicate therapy sessions. A client also can be advised to leave a phone message at a previously set time to describe how he or she is doing on completing the homework. These "check-ins" provide a boost of motivation to complete the homework between sessions. If homework compliance becomes a continuing difficulty, scheduling more therapy sessions may reduce the need for as much homework. That is, the time between therapy sessions can be reduced so that the client is practicing more often.

4.5.3   Adapting Treatment for Comorbidities

People with GAD often present with other comorbid problems. There is no research on the best way to treat people with GAD who have other diagnoses.

Some treatment outcome studies include people with comorbid GAD and other anxiety conditions. The outcome of these studies has not been found to be affected by the presence of this comorbidity. It is thought that GAD and depression are closely linked (as evidenced by the high comorbidity between the two conditions). Thus, treatment for GAD might also be enhanced by including some of the strategies for treating depression (e.g., Rehm, 2010).

Treatment should focus first on the most significant problem followed by secondary problems. Thus, a person with a primary diagnosis of social phobia and a secondary diagnosis of GAD might be best treated with the procedures that are effective in the treatment for social anxiety first (e.g., Antony & Rowa, 2008). However, concurrent treatment may be conducted on both problems depending on the impairment stemming from each problem. Thus, an assessment of functional impairment of each disorder is very important in the assessment.

4.6   Adapting Treatment for Different Age Groups

4.6.1   Children and Adolescents

Although younger children can show signs of excessive worry, children usually develop GAD when they are around 12 years old. Treatment for children and adolescents with GAD is similar in nature to treatment with adults. However, the content of treatment is provided at a level that is easier to understand. The cognitive component of treatment for children with GAD emphasizes positive "self-talk" rather than negative self-talk. Parents are often included in treatment to provide reinforcement and rewards for children's success and to learn to implement and practice the skills with their children.

Many treatments of anxiety disorders in youth are nonspecific to any particular anxiety disorder. However, these treatments often consist of the common CBT techniques described previously. It is important that these treatments are delivered with flexibility so that they can be applied across a variety of anxiety and other associated disorders. A thorough discussion of the treatment is outside the scope of this book. Some potential useful treatments for children can be found in the Further Reading section (e.g., Kendall & Hedtke, 2006; Pincus, Ehrenreich, & Spiegel, 2008).

4.6.2   Older Adults

There is some evidence that the incidence of GAD is bimodal, with the disorder most frequently occurring for people in younger ages (Wittchen et al., 1994) and older ages. Older adults who have GAD may be more likely to seek treatment from a primary care provider rather than a mental health service provider. Most treatment with older adults has been modified from currently existing treatment protocols for younger individuals. These treatments have similar outcomes to traditional GAD treatments (e.g., Hendriks, Oude Voshaar, Keijsers, Hoogduin, & van Balkom, 2008; Stanley et al., 2009).

When treating older adults, several factors need to be taken into account (see review by Ayers, Sorrell, Thorp, & Wetherell, 2007). For example, medical issues can complicate the assessment and treatment of anxiety in an older population. Many of the physical symptoms experienced in GAD can be similar to medical symptoms caused by medical illness. In addition, memory loss may make it difficult for some people to complete cognitive-based assignments. Memory aids (i.e., written reminders) and telephone calls can enhance treatment outcome (Mohlman et al., 2003). These memory aids may also enhance treatment compliance and motivation for treatment.

4.7   Adapting Treatment for Different Cultures

There is evidence that GAD occurs across different cultures (e.g., Martin, 2003). However, it is not known how GAD presents differently across cultures or which factors play more or less significant roles.

Very little research exists on how or whether treatment for GAD should be adapted for particular cultures. Therapists should be knowledgeable about how culture affects the symptoms that may be associated with GAD. Treatment providers must also be willing to explore how culture affects treatment. For example, in some cultural groups, people might expect a more direct approach to treatment, whereas others might appreciate a client-centered approach. The therapist should explore cultural differences and not assume that everyone from a particular culture fits a particular stereotype. That said, the therapist must continually pay attention to those behaviors and thoughts that may be influenced by culture (see American Psychological Association [APA], 2003, for multicultural guidelines for practice; see Bernal & Saez-Santiago, 2006; Griner & Smith, 2006, for discussions about the importance of culturally adapted treatments).

Case Vignette

This chapter describes a case example of an individual with GAD, along with a treatment plan. Treatment lasted for 12 sessions. The client experienced a reduction in symptoms as evidenced by lower scores on self-report symptom questionnaires.

Case Vignette: Laura's Worry

Laura, a 36-year-old mother of two children and an administrative assistant, presented with concerns about worrying too much. Her worry reportedly was causing difficulties in sleeping, muscle tension, and difficulties in getting her work completed. She came to treatment because "I am worrying that I worry too much."

The clinician conducted a structured clinical interview using the Anxiety Disorders Interview Schedule for DSM-IV. Laura indicated a significant amount of distress and impairment with regard to GAD. She also indicated some mild depression symptoms, but not enough to qualify for a major depressive episode or major depressive disorder.

Assessment

On the Worry Domains Questionnaire, Laura indicated significant levels of worry across many domains (obtaining a total score of 97 out of 125). Her score of 74 on the Penn State Worry Questionnaire was very similar to the mean of a clinical sample of people with GAD. Similarly, she self-reported having many of the criteria of GAD on the Worry and Anxiety Questionnaire.

Laura indicated a high level of intolerance of uncertainty as measured by the Intolerance of Uncertainty Scale (score of 84). She also indicated many positive beliefs about worry as assessed by the Why Worry Scale and the Consequences of Worry Scale. She indicated some reluctance to experience negative internal states as evidenced by the Acceptance and Action Questionnaire. Additionally, she indicated worry about worry on the Meta-Worry Questionnaire.

Laura's self-reported depression was in the mild range (z score of -1.5 compared with a clinical group). Her stress score was in the moderate range and her anxiety score was in the mild range.

Below is an example of a conversation with the therapist during the assessment. It illustrates one of Laura's worries and how she attempts to avoid thinking about her situation too deeply. It also demonstrates her tendency to jump from worry to worry.

Therapist: Tell me something that you worried about recently.

Client: Last night, the phone rang at 10:00. The phone really causes me to worry a lot, but someone calling that late makes me think that something bad has happened. It was actually a wrong number, but it made me start worry about my Mom. I have been worried that she is getting older. She turned 62 in July.

Therapist: So when the phone rang, what was your worry about your mother?

Client: The ringing of the phone startled me. It got me thinking that something might have happened to my Mom. I started to worry about her. I worry because she has fallen in the past, and I think she might fall and break a hip or something. Or maybe she might get sick … or get cancer. I worry about all of these things.

Therapist: What do you picture happening if your mom did pass away?

Client: Well … I don't even know. I don't even want to think about that. It gets me really anxious. I would rather think about something else. I wouldn't even know what to do. I would have so many responsibilities.…

Psychoeducation and Treatment Conceptualization Discussion

Following her assessment, the clinician and Laura discussed treatment options and her case conceptualization (see Figure 7). The client agreed that her worry was excessive, and she wanted treatment. Laura and her therapist agreed that weekly sessions would be best based on Laura's schedule. A discussion of the general format of treatment was discussed (e.g., length of sessions, homework) and psychoeducation about GAD began. A big part of the psychoeducation was to discuss Laura's case conceptualization (see Figure 7). Part of the discussion about how different factors maintained Laura's high amount of worry is presented below.

Therapist: Jumping from worry to worry can reduce anxiety in the short run but may actually be maintaining your anxiety over the long run. That is, by not fully imagining how the worry could unfold, you are actually getting rid of the anxiety like an aspirin gets rid of a headache. However, there is a consequence of trying to get rid of the anxiety – it actually makes the worry seem much worse than it truly is. That is, you never see that you could handle the situation because you never let yourself fully imagine it. That said, it is quite natural and understandable to want to get rid of the anxiety.

[…]

Therapist: Worry can help us prepare for future danger or threat. It helps us to figure out what we can do to fix the situation. There are several factors that maintain excessive worry. One is the tendency to try to distract yourself from worrying without feeling as though you've resolved anything in your mind. Worrying through one situation completely can lead us to come up with a variety of solutions. When we don't allow ourselves to think things through

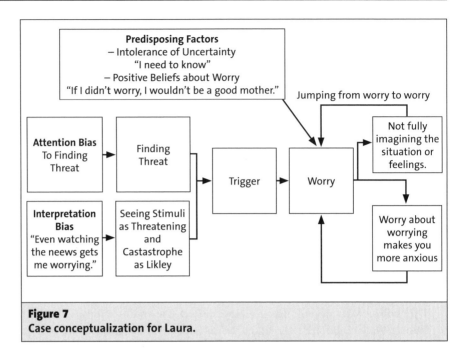

Figure 7
Case conceptualization for Laura.

and to imagine our worst possible fears coming true, worry can spiral into increased worry and anxiety. Do you ever find yourself trying to think about something else when you start worrying?

Cognitive Components of Treatment

Following the psychoeducation portions of treatment, the therapist explained thoughts and how they affect Laura's worry. A transcript of some of that discussion is presented below.

Therapist: Thoughts are instrumental in affecting emotions like anxiety. The key question to ask yourself is whether your judgment of risk is true. Or is this worry really likely or probable? For the most part, people with excessive worry overestimate the likelihood that their worry will come true. We are going to challenge the worries and anxious thoughts when they are out of proportion with the actual risk. Thinking is often an automatic process, so it may be difficult at first to identify these thoughts when you're anxious. Let's look at one of your worries you mentioned, the one that your daughter might get hurt ice-skating. What specifically were you worried about?

Client: That she would get seriously hurt. She skates so fast and now she is skating with a male partner. So not only is she at risk of falling, but now she is supposed to be tossed and spun by her partner.

Therapist: How specifically do you imagine your daughter getting hurt?

Client: Probably a broken neck. Something that will result in paralysis or death. It has happened before.

Therapist: What injuries have happened to your daughter previously?

Client: Nothing, really. She has jammed her fingers and gotten scratched a bit falling on the ice. But it is so slippery, and she moves so fast.

Therapist: So what you're saying is that you had predicted that she would be injured during the game, but it hasn't happen. When we're anxious, we tend to overestimate the probability of a bad occurrence. While you are feeling anxious and worried, what is the probability in your mind that your daughter would be hurt, from 0 to 100%?

Client: About 50%.

Therapist: So that means that for every two times that your daughter ice skates, she gets hurt once. Is that correct?

Client: Umm, no, I don't think it's that high. Maybe about 25%.

Therapist: To counter the tendency to overestimate the chances of negative future events, it is helpful to ask yourself what evidence supports your anxious belief. What evidence can you provide from your daughter's skating history to account for your belief that she will get hurt in one out of every four times?

Client: Well, none. But it can always happen

Therapist: What are other alternatives to your daughter getting seriously hurt?

Client: She could get a minor injury, like a sprained ankle or something of that nature.

Therapist: Right. And what would be the probability of your daughter getting a minor versus a major injury?

Client: Probably higher.

Therapist: To go back to your original worry, what would you rate the probability of your daughter getting seriously injured?

Client: Low, about 5%. So it is silly for me to think these irrational thoughts.

Therapist: When anxious, it is quite natural to focus on the more negative possibilities in order to prepare for them should they come true.

Client: I can now see that there isn't as high of a chance of my daughter becoming paralyzed, but it is still possible.

Therapist: There's always that possibility, however minute. However, every time you tell yourself "it is still possible," you are basically throwing out all the evidence disconfirming that belief. Worrying about a future event does nothing to change its probability of occurring. It only makes you feel even more anxious.

Acceptance of Intolerance of Uncertainty

Therapist: Let's talk a bit about intolerance of uncertainty, which is a fuel for worry. People who are intolerant of uncertainty don't like those situations when they don't know the outcome. The more the person is intolerant of uncertainty, the more that person is likely to ask "what if" questions. People who are intolerant of uncertainty may also notice uncertainty faster than other people. Let me give an example, a person who is intolerant of uncertainty might immediately think about all possible problems when planning a vacation, even though there is a small chance of any of those problems occurring. That is, people who are intolerant of uncertainty recognize uncertainty very quickly, and they think about all the potential bad things that could result from it. What do you do to deal with "uncertain" situations?

Client: I don't know. I never really thought about it. I can't think of anything.

Therapist: Some people I have worked with have said they might ask for reassurance from their friends and families before making any decision.

Client: I definitely do that. I ask my Dad about everything. This sometime bothers my husband, but he won't give me that reassurance that my Dad gives.

Therapist: Because intolerance of uncertainty is something that seems to fuel GAD, let's think about ways that we could change it and see whether it applies to you. First, let's break the term into the two parts: intolerance and uncertainty. We could decrease worrying by either increasing our certainty or decreasing our intolerance. That is, if we increased our certainty, then we would not feel the need to worry because we would know the outcome of every situation. On the other hand, if we decreased our intolerance or need to know, then we would not need to worry as much either. People with GAD tend to do a lot of trying to increase certainty, usually by worrying about things....

Therapist: Uncertainty is unavoidable. Everyone has some amount of uncertainty in their life that they cannot get rid of. We can't be certain that we will have a job, good health, or good relationships. Do you think it is possible that we can be absolutely certain?

Client: It isn't possible. I think I have been trying so hard to find the answer, but in the end I just have to accept that I can't find the answer to everything.

Therapist: Great. So we need to find a way to decrease your need to know. Sometimes this is easier said than done.

Client: I agree. I wanted to ask you how I change my need to know. I think I have a lot of habits that would be hard to break.

Therapist: We are going to practice some behaviors so that you can learn to accept uncertainty rather than immediately acting to do something to get rid of it. Some of these skills will be acting as if we don't mind uncertainty. That is, when we see those situations we will act as if we don't care about the uncertainty. We will just notice the thoughts of uncertainty and behave as if we don't mind them.

Worry Exposure

The next component of treatment focuses on worry exposure as a means to assist Laura in fully processing her worries. Below is a transcript of some of the therapy that was completed.

Therapist: Today we are going to work on worry exposure. We discussed how worrying is usually an attempt to problem solve future threatening or dangerous situations. For people who worry excessively, the worry can jump from one worry to another. This type of worrying gets in the way of problem solving. Additionally, the individual focuses on negative predictions that then increase anxiety. The worry exposure will help you gain a sense of control over these worries, and will also help you to manage them a bit more productively. One idea for why these worries persist is because you might not be thinking about them completely. That is, you may not be processing or thinking through the worry completely. For example, when a particularly scary worry comes to mind, sometimes people will try to distract themselves. They might also be saying to themselves, "I can't think about this," because the thoughts cause so much anxiety. It is quite normal to not want to think about something that upsets you. However, as we talked about before, avoiding thinking about it can make it worse in the long run.... I'm going to ask you to think about a worry for at least 30 minutes a day. You'll do nothing but think about this worry as vividly as possible for 30 minutes. Although this time may sound overwhelming, we're actually attempting to reduce the amount of time that you're worrying from 80% of the day to around 30 minutes a day.

Let's practice this with a worry you mentioned last week. You described a situation in which you were worried when your daughter had a friend over to the house. What is the very worst image that you can envision when your child brings a friend over?

Client: She'll probably think I am a bad mother because my floors are dirty. Just thinking about that reminds me I have to get my vacuum fixed.... She will see my dirty floors and cluttered counter. She'll probably go home and tell her mother that I'm not a good mother. I'll lose everyone's respect, and everyone will be laughing at me.

Therapist: How well do you see the scene right now? Rate it on a scale from 0 to 10, where 10 means that is the imagined scene feels like real life and you can see it perfectly, and 0 means you can't really imagine it at all.

Client: About 5.

Therapist: Maybe you can imagine it as if it were a movie. I want you to picture your daughter's friend looking around at the floors and the clutter. Picture her facial expressions. Picture yourself in that situation watching her look around, just knowing that she will soon tell her mother about your messy house. How vivid is that image?

Client: Clearer. About a 7.

Therapist: Good. Now keep imagining that scene for the next few minutes. Play it out over and over again in your head. Make it as vivid as possible as if you can see and touch everything in the scene....

[Therapist and client imagine the scene for 30 minutes.]

Therapist: Now, I want you to begin to challenge your thoughts in order to counter that image in your mind.

Client: Well, I guess that my daughter's friend may not even care about the house. She might be so into talking with my daughter that she wouldn't even notice. I try to think about when I was her age and I don't think I thought about those things so much. Even if she did notice, it is probably not guaranteed that she would go home and tell her mother. And if she did tell her mother, it probably doesn't matter. Although I don't like people to think bad things about me, I can't be perfect to everyone.

Therapist: Excellent. How is your anxiety level now?

Client: Very low, maybe a 15. I don't know about doing this at home. I didn't really like it, and without you here I think I would have found something else to do to distract myself. It is uncomfortable.

Therapist: Maybe you can tell me again why we do the worry exposure?

Client: By doing it I am facing the thoughts I usually avoid. If I do it enough, I will have less anxiety in reaction to those thoughts. It is like you said with getting a vaccine. By doing it I am building up my immune system for future worries.

Therapist: Great explanation. And it *will* probably be a bit uncomfortable, but just as it did here, the discomfort goes away with time. Do you think you want to try this at home?

Relapse Prevention

Therapist: As treatment is ending soon, we should review your skills. As we discussed in the beginning, the goal is for you to become your own therapist. Importantly, once treatment ends, you will need to keep practicing all the skills that we learned in session. We should also discuss setbacks. Sometimes people with GAD start to worry more frequently, which makes them think they have "relapsed." Thinking "I've relapsed" makes one feel that they can do nothing to change what is happening. Rather, we like to think about times of increased worry as a setback or even a learning experience. Moreover, it is quite likely that you will have periods of ups and downs, times when you worry more or less. However, you will not necessarily relapse to the point where you were when you began therapy. Rather, you can frame the times when you worry more, the down periods, as setbacks. When you have a setback, it is actually a great time to evaluate what happened and what you might have done to make the situation better or worse. When perceived this way, the setback can be seen as a learning experience.

Progress and Treatment Outcome

Laura underwent posttreatment and follow-up assessments, each of which entailed administration of the ADIS-IV and self-report questionnaires. Following treatment and across the follow-up period, Laura continued to experience decreasing levels of anxiety and worry. In addition, Laura indicated she felt more in control of her worry and anxiety. Laura reported that she still experienced some worry during the day, but when she did worry she was able to handle it by facing it rather than distracting herself.

6

Further Reading

Antony, M. M., & Rowa, K. P. (2008). *Social anxiety disorder* . Cambridge, MA: Hogrefe & Huber.
  This book is an excellent clinician resource on social anxiety disorder, which is a common comorbid condition seen with GAD.
Arkowitz, H., Westra, H. A., & Rollnick, S. (2007). *Motivational interviewing in the treatment of psychological problems* (1st ed.). New York, NY: Guilford Press.
  This volume gives practical advice on how to conduct motivational interviewing for common psychological problems.
Butler, G., Fennell, M., & Hackmann, A. (2008). *Cognitive-behavioral therapy for anxiety disorders: Mastering clinical challenges* (1st ed.). New York, NY: Guilford Press.
  This volume provides an excellent resource for case conceptualization of anxiety disorders. It has multiple diagrams which can be very useful in presenting the case conceptualization to the client.
Kendall, P. C., & Hedtke, K. A. (2006). *Cognitive-behavioral therapy for anxious children: Therapist manual, Third Edition* (3rd ed.). Ardmore, PA: Workbook Publishing.
  This treatment manual for children has proven to be transportable and adaptable to other countries/cultures.
Pincus, D. B., Ehrenreich, J. T., & Spiegel, D. A. (2008). *Riding the wave workbook (workbook).* New York, NY: Oxford University Press.
  This workbook for adolescents is very helpful in the treatment of GAD.
Rehm, L. P. (2010). *Advances in Psychotherapy – Evidence-Based Practice: Depression.* Cambridge, MA: Hogrefe Publishing.
  Excellent clinician resource on depression, a common comorbid condition
Roemer, L., & Orsillo, S. M. (2002). Expanding our conceptualization of and treatment for generalized anxiety disorder: Integrating mindfulness/acceptance-based approaches with existing cognitive-behavioral models. *Clinical Psychology: Science and Practice, 9*(1), 54–68. doi:10.1093/clipsy.9.1.54
  This article describes some of the background of acceptance-based treatment in more detail.
Zinbarg, R. E., Craske, M. G., & Barlow, D. H. (2006). *Mastery of your anxiety and worry (MAW): Client workbook* (2nd ed.). New York, NY: Oxford University Press.
  This client workbook can be helpful in assisting the client by having them read through the chapters.

7

References

Alden, L. E., Wiggins, J. S., & Pincus, A. L. (1990). Construction of Circumplex Scales for the Inventory of Interpersonal Problems. *Journal of Personality Assessment, 55,* 521–536. doi:10.1207/s15327752jpa5503&4_10

American Psychiatric Association. (1980). *Diagnostic and statistical manual of mental disorders* (3th ed.). Washington, DC: Author.

American Psychiatric Association. (1987). *Diagnostic and statistical manual of mental disorders* (3th ed., revised). Washington, DC: Author.

American Psychiatric Association. (1994). *Diagnostic and statistical manual of mental disorders* (4th ed.). Washington, DC: Author.

American Psychiatric Association. (2000). *Diagnostic and statistical manual of mental disorders* (4th ed., text revision). Washington, DC: Author.

American Psychiatric Association. (2010). *Proposed changes to the Diagnostic and Statistical Manual of Mental Disorders.* Retrieved from http://www.dsm5.org/ProposedRevisions/Pages/proposedrevision.aspx?rid=167

American Psychological Association. (2003). Guidelines on multicultural education, training, research, practice and organizational change for psychologists. *American Psychologist, 58,* 377–402.

Amir, N., Beard, C., Burns, M., & Bomyea, J. (2009). Attention modification program in individuals with generalized anxiety disorder. *Journal of Abnormal Psychology, 118,* 28–33.

Anderson, J. M., & Palm, M. E. (2006). Pharmacological treatments for worry: Focus on generalized anxiety disorder. In G. C. L. Davey & A. Wells (Eds.), *Worry and its psychological disorders: Theory, assessment and treatment* (pp. 305–334). West Sussex, England: Wiley.

Antony, M. M., Orsillo, S. M., & Roemer, L. (2001). *Practitioner's guide to empirically based measures of anxiety (AABT Clinical Assessment)* (1st ed.). New York, NY: Springer.

Antony, M. M., & Rowa, K. P. (2008). *Social anxiety disorder* . Cambridge, MA: Hogrefe & Huber.

Arkowitz, H., Westra, H. A., Miller, W. R., & Rollnick, S. (2008). *Motivational interviewing in the treatment of psychological problems.* New York, NY: Guilford Press.

Ayers, C. R., Sorrell, J. T., Thorp, S. R., & Wetherell, J. L. (2007). Evidence-based psychological treatments for late-life anxiety. *Psychology and Aging, 22,* 8–17. doi:10.1037/0882-7974.22.1.8.

Barlow, D. H. (1988). *Anxiety and its disorders: The nature and treatment of anxiety and panic.* New York, NY: Guilford Press.

Barlow, D. H., Rapee, R. M., & Brown, T. A. (1992). Behavioral treatment of generalized anxiety disorder. *Behavior Therapy, 23,* 551–570.

Barmish, A. J., & Kendall, P. C. (2005). Should parents be co-clients in cognitive-behavioral therapy for anxious youth? *Journal of Clinical Child & Adolescent Psychology, 34,* 569–581. doi:10.1207/s15374424jccp3403_12

Barrett, J. E., Barrett, J. A., Oxman, T. E., & Gerber, P. D., (1988). The prevalence of psychiatric disorders in primary car practice. *Archives of General Psychiatry, 45,* 1100–1106.

Beck, A. T., Steer, R. A., & Brown, G. K. (1996). *Manual for Beck Depression Inventory II (BDI-II).* San Antonio, TX: Psychology Corporation.

Behar, E., Alcaine, O., Zuellig, A. R., & Borkovec, T. D. (2003). Screening for generalized anxiety disorder using the Penn State Worry Questionnaire: A receiver operating characteristic analysis. *Journal of Behavior Therapy and Experimental Psychiatry, 34,* 25–43. doi:10.1016/S0005-7916(03)00004-1

Behar, E., DiMarco, I. D., Hekler, E. B., Mohlman, J., & Staples, A. M. (2009). Current theoretical models of generalized anxiety disorder (GAD): Conceptual review and treatment implications. *Journal of Anxiety Disorders, 23,* 1011–1023. doi:10.1016/j.janxdis.2009.07.006

Bernal, G., & Saez-Santiago, E. (2006). Culturally centered psychosocial interventions. *Journal of Community Psychology, 34,* 121–132.

Blazer, D. G., Hughes, D. C., George, L. K. (1987). The epidemiology of depression in an elderly community population. *Gerontologist, 27,* 281–287.

Blazer, D. G., Hughes, D. C., George, L. K., Swartz, M., & Boyer, R. (1991). Generalized anxiety disorder. In L. N. Robins & D. A. Regier (Eds.), *Psychiatric disorders in America: The Epidemiologic Catchment Area Study* (pp. 180–203). New York, NY: Free Press.

Bond, F. W., Hayes, S. C., Baer, R. A., Carpenter, K. M., Orcutt, H. K., Waltz, T., & Zettle, R.D. (2011). *Preliminary psychometric properties of the Acceptance and Action Questionnaire – II: A revised measure of psychological flexibility and acceptance.* Manuscript submitted for publication.

Borkovec, T. D., & Costello, E., (1993). Efficacy of applied relaxation and cognitive behavioral therapy in the treatment of generalized anxiety disorder. *Journal of Consulting and Clinical Psychology, 61,* 611–619.

Borkovec, T. D., & Inz, J. (1990). The effect of worry on cardiovascular response to phobic imagery. *Beahaviour Research and Therapy, 28,* 69–73.

Borkovec, T. D., Newman, M. G., & Castonguay, L. G. (2004). Cognitive-behavioral therapy for generalized anxiety disorder with integrations from interpersonal and experiential therapies. *Focus, 2,* 392–401.

Borkovec, T. D., Newman, M. G., Pincus, A. L., & Lytle, R. (2002). A component analysis of cognitive-behavioral therapy for generalized anxiety disorder and the role of interpersonal problems. *Journal of Consulting and Clinical Psychology, 70,* 288–298. doi:10.1037/0022-006X.70.2.288

Borkovec, T. D., Robinson, E., Pruzinsky, T., & Depree, J. (1983). Preliminary exploration of worry: Some characteristics and processes. *Behaviour Research and Therapy, 21,* 9–16.

Borkovec, T. D., & Roemer, L. (1995). Perceived functions of worry among generalized anxiety disorder subjects: Distraction from more emotionally distressing topics? *Journal of Behavior Therapy and Experimental Psychiatry, 26,* 25–30.

Borkovec, T. D., & Ruscio, A. M. (2001). Psychotherapy for generalized anxiety disorder. *Journal of Clinical Psychiatry, 62,* 37–45.

Borkovec, T. D., Shadick, R., & Hopkins, M. (1991). The nature of normal and pathological worry. In R. Rapee & D. H. Barlow (Eds.), *Chronic anxiety: Generalized anxiety disorder and mixed anxiety-depression* (pp. 29–51). New York, NY: Guilford Press.

Breitholz, E., Johansson, B., & Ost, L. G. (1999). Cognitions in generalized anxiety disorder and panic disorder patients: A prospective approach. *Behaviour Research and Therapy, 37,* 533–544.

Brown, T. A., Antony, M. M., & Barlow, D. H. (1992). Psychometric properties of the Penn State Worry Questionnaire in a clinical anxiety disorders sample. *Behaviour Research and Therapy, 30,* 33–38.

Brown, T. A., Barlow, D. H., & Liebowitz, M. R. (1994). The empirical basis of generalized anxiety disorder. *American Journal of Psychiatry, 151,* 1272–1280.

Brown, T., Di Nardo, P., & Barlow, D. (1994). *Anxiety Disorders Interview Schedule for DSM-IV (ADIS-IV).* Albany, NY: Graywind.

Brown, T., Di Nardo, P., Lehman, C. L., & Campbell, L. A. (2001). Reliability of *DSM-IV* anxiety and mood disorders: Implications for the classification of emotional disorders. *Journal of Abnormal Psychology, 110,* 49–58.

Butler, G., Fennell, M., & Hackmann, A. (2008). *Cognitive-behavioral therapy for anxiety disorders: Mastering clinical challenges* (1st ed.). New York, NY: Guilford Press.

Butler, G., Fennell, M., Robson, P., & Gelder, M. (1991). Comparison of behavior therapy and cognitive behavior therapy in the treatment of generalized anxiety disorder. *Journal of Consulting and Clinical Psychology, 59,* 167–175.

Butler, G., Gelder, M., Hibbert, G., Cullington, A., & Klimes, I. (1987). Anxiety management: Developing effective strategies. *Behavior Research and Therapy, 25,* 517–522.

Butler, G., & Matthews, A. (1987). Anticipatory anxiety and risk perception. *Cognitive Therapy and Research, 11,* 551–565.

Campbell, L. A., & Brown, T. A. (2002). Generalized anxiety disorder. In M. M. Antony & D. H. Barlow (Eds.), *Handbook of assessment and treatment planning for psychological disorders* (pp. 147–181). New York, NY: Guilford Press.

Carter, R. M., Wittchen, H. U., Pfister, H., & Kessler, R. C. (2001). One-year prevalence of subthreshold and threshold DSM-IV generalized anxiety disorder in a nationally representative sample. *Depression and Anxiety, 13,* 78–88.

Cartwright-Hatton, S., & Wells, A. (1997). Beliefs about worry and intrusions: The Meta-Cognitions Questionnaire and its correlates. *Journal of Anxiety Disorders, 11,* 279–296.

Covin, R., Dozois, D. J. A., & Westra, H. A. (2008). An evaluation of the psychometric properties of the consequences of worry scale (COWS). *Cognitive Therapy Research, 32,* 133–142.

Covin, R., Ouimet, A. J., Seeds, P. M., & Dozois, D. J. A. (2008). A meta-analysis of CBT for pathological worry among clients with GAD. *Journal of Anxiety Disorders, 22,* 108–116.

Craske, M. G., & Barlow, D. H. (2006). *Mastery of your anxiety and worry: Workbook (Treatments that work)* (2nd ed.). New York, NY: Oxford University Press.

Davey, C. L., Tallis, F., & Capuzzo, N. (1996). Beliefs about the consequences of worrying. *Cognitive Therapy and Research, 20,* 499–520.

Diefenbach, G. J., Stanley, M. A., & Beck, J. G. (2001). Worry content reported by older adults with and without generalized anxiety disorder. *Aging and Mental Health, 5,* 269–274.

Dugas, M. J., Buhr, K., & Ladouceur, R. (2005). The role of intolerance of uncertainty in etiology and maintenance. In R. G. Heimberg, C. L. Turk, & D. S. Mennin (Eds.), *Generalized anxiety disorders: Advances in research and practice* (pp. 164–186). New York, NY: Guilford Press.

Dugas, M. J., Freeston, M. H., Provencher, M. D., Lachance, S., Ladouceur, R., & Gosselin, P. (2001). Le Questionnaire sur l'inquiétude et l'anxiété: Validation dans des échantillons non cliniques et cliniques [The Worry and Anxiety Questionnaire: Validation among nonclinical and clinical samples]. *Journal de Thérapie Comportementale et Cognitive, 11,* 31–36.

Dugas, M. J., Gagnon, F., Ladouceur, R., & Freeston, M. H. (1998). Generalized anxiety disorder: A preliminary test of a conceptual model. *Behavior Research and Therapy, 36,* 215–226.

Dugas, M. J., Gosselin, P., & Ladouceur, R. (2001). Intolerance of uncertainty and worry: Investigating narrow specificity in a nonclinical sample. *Cognitive Therapy and Research, 25,* 551–558.

Dugas, M. J., & Ladouceur, R. (2000). Treatment of Gad: Targeting intolerance of uncertainty in two types of worry. *Behavior Modification, 24,* 635–657.

Dugas, M. J., Ladouceur, R., Leger, E., Freeston, M. H., & Provencher, M. D., Boisvert, J. M. (2003). Group cognitive-behavioral therapy for generalized anxiety disorder: Treatment outcome and long-term follow-up. *Journal of Consulting and Clinical Psychology, 71,* 821–825.

Dugas, M. J., Marchand, A., & Ladouceur, R. (2005). Further validation of a cognitive-behavioral model of generalized anxiety disorder: Diagnostic and symptom specificity. *Journal of Anxiety Disorders, 19,* 329–343.

Dugas, M. J., & Robichaud, M. (2007). *Cognitive-behavioral treatment for generalized anxiety disorder: From science to practice.* New York, NY: Routledge.

Dugas, M. J., Savard, P., Gaudet, A., Turcotte, J., Laugesen, N., Robichaud, M., & Koerner, N. (2007). Can the components of a cognitive model predict the severity of generalized anxiety disorder? *Behavior Therapy, 38,* 169–178.

Eysenck, M. W., MacLeod, C., & Mathews, A. (1987). Cognitive functioning and anxiety. *Psychological Research, 49,* 189–195.

Eysenck, M. W., Mogg, K., May, J., Richards, A., & Mathews, A. (1991). Bias in interpretation of ambiguous sentences related to threat in anxiety. *Journal of Abnormal Psychology, 100,* 144–150.

Fairburn, C. G. (2008). *Cognitive behavior therapy and eating disorders.* New York, NY: Guilford Press.

First, M., Spitzer, R., Gibbon, M., Williams, J. (2002). *Structured clinical interview for axis I disorders, patient edition.* New York: Biometrics Research, New York State Psychiatric Institute.

Foa, E. B., & Kozak, M. J. (1986). Emotional processing of fear: Exposure to corrective information. *Psychological Bulletin, 99,* 20–35.

Freeston, M. H., Rheaume, J., Letarte, H., Dugas, M., & Ladouceur, R. (1994). Why do people worry? *Personality and Individual Differences, 17,* 791–802.

Galenberg, A. J., Lydiard, R. B., Rudolph, R. L., Aguiar, L., Haskins, J. T., & Salinas, E. (2000). Efficacy of venlafaxine extended-release capsules in nondepressed outpatients with generalized anxiety disorder: A 6-month randomized controlled trial. *JAMA, 283,* 3082–3088.

Ginsburg, G. S., & Schlossberg, M. C. (2002). Family-based treatment of childhood anxiety disorders. *International Review of Psychiatry, 14,* 143–154. doi:10.1080/09540260220132662

Goodman, W. K., Price, L. H., Rasmussen, S. A., Mazure, C., Fleischmann, R. L., Hill, C. L., ... Charney, D. S. (1989). The Yale-Brown Obsessive Compulsive Scale, I: Development, use, and reliability. *Archives of General Psychiatry, 46,* 1006–1011.

Gould, R. A., Safren, S. A., Washington, D. O., & Otto, M. W. (2004). A meta-analytic review of cognitive-behavioral treatments. In R. G. Heimberg, C. L. Turk, & D. S. Mennin (Eds.), *Generalized anxiety disorders: Advances in research and practice* (pp. 248–264). New York, NY: Guilford Press.

Griner, D., & Smith, T. (2006). Culturally adapted mental health interventions: A meta-analytic review. *Psychotherapy: Theory, Research, Practice, Training, 43,* 531–548.

Hayes, S. A., Hirsch, C. R., Krebs, G., & Mathews, A. (2010). The effects of modifying interpretation bias on worry in generalized anxiety disorder. *Behavior Research, and Therapy, 48,* 171–178.

Hayes, S. C., & Ju, W. (1998). Rule-governed behavior. In W. O'Donahue (Ed.), *Learning and behavior therapy* (pp. 374–381). Boston, MA: Allyn and Bacon.

Hayes, S. A., Orsillo, S. M., & Roemer, L. (2010). Changes in proposed mechanisms of action during an acceptance-based behavior therapy for generalized anxiety disorder. *Behaviour Research and Therapy, 48,* 238–245. doi:10.1016/j.brat.2009.11.006

Hayes, S. C., Strosahl, K. D., & Wilson, K. G. (1999). *Acceptance and commitment therapy: An experiential approach to behavior change.* New York, NY: Guilford Press.

Hayes, S. C., Strosahl, K. D., Wilson, K. G., Bissett, R. T., Pistorello, J., Toarmino, D., ... McCurry, S. M. (2004). Measuring experiential avoidance: A preliminary test of a working model. *The Psychological Record, 54,* 553–578.

Hayes, S. C., Wilson, K. G., Gifford, E. V., Follette, V. M., & Strosahl, K. (1996). Experiential avoidance and behavioral disorders: A functional dimensional approach to diagnosis and treatment. *Journal of Consulting and Clinical Psychology, 64,* 1152–1168.

Hendriks, G. J., Oude Voshaar, R. C., Keijsers, G. P. J., Hoogduin, C. A. L., & van Balkom, A. J. L. M. (2008). Cognitive-behavioural therapy for late-life anxiety disorders: a systematic review and meta-analysis. *Acta Psychiatrica Scandinavica, 117*(6), 403–411. doi:10.1111/j.1600-0447.2008.01190.x

Hirsch, C. R., MacLeod, C, Mathews, A., Sandher, O., Siyani, A., Hayes, S. (2010). The contribution of attentional bias to worry: Distinguishing the roles of selective engagement and disengagement. *Journal of Anxiety Disorders, 25,* 272–277. doi: 10.1016/j. janxdis.2010.09.013

Inner Health Studio. *Free relaxation script: Progressive muscle relaxation exercise.* Retrieved from http://www.innerhealthstudio.com/progressive-muscle-relaxation-exercise.html.

Joormann, J., & Stober, J. (1997). Measuring facets of worry: A LISREL analysis of the Worry Domains Questionnaire. *Personality and Individual Differences, 23,* 827–837.

Kabat-Zinn, J. (1994). *Wherever you go there you are.* New York, NY: Hyperion.

Kabat-Zinn, J., Massion, A. O., Kristeller, J., Peterson, L. G., Fletcher, K. E., Pbert, L., ... Santorelli, S. F. (1992). Effectiveness of a meditation-based stress reduction program in the treatment of anxiety disorders. *American Journal of Psychiatry, 149,* 936–943.

Kendall, P. C., & Hedtke, K. A. (2006). *Cognitive-behavioral therapy for anxious children: Therapist manual* (3rd ed.). Asdmore, PA: Workbook.

Ladouceur, R., Dugas, M. J., Freeston, M. H., Leger, E., Gagnon, F., & Thibodeau, N. (2000). Efficacy of a cognitive-behavioral treatment for generalized anxiety disorder: Evaluation in a controlled clinical trial. *Journal of Consulting and Clinical Psychology, 68,* 957–964.

Ladouceur, R., Dugas, M. J., Freeston, M. H., Rheaume, J., Blais, F., Boisvert, J. M., ... Thibodeau, N. (1999). Specificity of generalized anxiety disorder symptoms and processes. *Behavior Therapy, 30,* 191–207.

Lovibond, S. H., & Lovibond, P. F. (1995). *Manual for the Depression Anxiety Stress Scales.* (2nd ed.) Sydney: Psychology Foundation.

Mancuso, D. M., Townsend, M. H., & Mercante, D. E., (1993). Long-term follow-up of generalized anxiety disorder. *Comprehensive Psychiatry, 34,* 441–446.

Martin, P. (2003). The epidemiology of anxiety disorders: A review. *Dialogues in Clinical Neuroscience, 5,* 281–298.

Mathews, A., Richards, A., & Eysenck, M. (1989). Interpretation of homophones related to threat in anxiety states. *Journal of Abnormal Psychology, 98,* 31–34.

Meyer, T. J., Miller, M. L., Metzger, R. L., & Borkovec, T. D. (1990). Development and validation of the Penn State Worry Questionnaire. *Behaviour Research and Therapy, 28,* 487–495.

Miller, W. R., & Rollnick, S. (2002). *Motivational interviewing: Preparing people for change* (2nd ed.). New York, NY: Guilford Press.

Mogg, K., & Bradley, B. (2005). Attentional bias in generalized anxiety disorder versus depressive disorder. *Cognitive Therapy and Research, 29*(1), 29–45. doi:10.1007/s10608-005-1646-y

Mogg, K., Bradley, B. P., Miller, T., & Potts, H. (1994). Interpretation of homophones related to threat: anxiety or response bias effects? *Cognitive Therapy and Research, 18,* 461–477.

Mohlman, J., Gorenstein, E. E., Kleber, M., de Jesus, M., Gorman, J. M., & Papp, L. A. (2003). Standard and enhanced cognitive-behavior therapy for late-life generalized anxiety disorder: two pilot investigations. *American Journal of Geriatric Psychiatry, 11,* 24–32.

Moller, H. J., Volz, Hp. P., Reimann, I. W., & Stoll, K.-D. (2001). Opipramol for the treatment of generalized anxiety disorder: A placebo-controlled trial including an alprazolam-treated group. *Journal of Clinical Psychopharmacology, 21,* 59–65.

Myers, K. M., & Davis, M. (2007). Mechanisms of fear extinction. *Molecular Psychiatry, 12,* 120–150.

National Institute of Mental Health. (2010). The numbers count: Mental disorders in America. Retrieved September 29, 2010, from www.nimh.nih.gov/health/publications/the-numbers-count-mental-disorders-in-america/index.shtml

Noyes, R., Holt, C. S., & Woodman, C. L. (1996). Natural course of anxiety disorders. In M. Mavissakalian & R. F. Prien (Eds.), *Long-term treatments of anxiety disorders* (pp. 1–48). Washington, DC: American Psychiatric Press.

Pincus, D. B., Ehrenreich, J. T., & Spiegel, D. A. (2008). *Riding the wave workbook* [Workbook]. New York, NY: Oxford University Press.

Power, K. G., Simpson, R. J., Swanson, V., Wallace, L. A., Feistner, A. T. C., & Sharp, D. (1990). A controlled comparison of cognitive-behaviour therapy, Diazepam, and placebo, alone and in combination, for the treatment of generalised anxiety disorder. *Journal of Anxiety Disorders, 4,* 267–292. doi:10.1016/0887-6185(90)90026-6

Prados, J. M. (2010). Do beliefs about the utility of worry facilitate worry? *Journal of Anxiety Disorders, 25,* 217–223. doi:10.1016/j.janxdis.2010.09.005

Purdon, C. (2000, July). *Metacognition and the persistence of worry.* Paper presented at the annual conference of the British Association of Behavioural and Cognitive Psychotherapy, London.

Quirk, G. J., & Mueller, D. (2008). Neural mechanisms of extinction learning and retrieval. *Neuropsychopharmacology, 33,* 56–72.

Rehm, L. P. (2010). *Depression.* Cambridge, MA: Hogrefe Publishing.

Rickels, K., Pollack, M. H., Sheehan, D., & Haskins, J. (2000). Efficacy of extended-release venlafaxine in nondepressed outpatients with generalized anxiety disorder. *American Journal of Psychiatry, 157,* 968–974.

Roemer, L., Molina, S., & Borkovec, T. D. (1997). An investigation of worry content among generally anxious individuals. *Journal of Nervous and Mental Disease, 185,* 314–319.

Roemer, L., Molina, S., Litz, B., & Borkovec, T. D. (1997). Preliminary investigation of the role of previous exposure to potentially traumatizing events in generalized anxiety disorder. *Depression and Anxiety, 4,* 134–138.

Roemer, L., & Orsillo, S. M. (2002). Expanding our conceptualization of and treatment for generalized anxiety disorder: Integrating mindfulness/acceptance-based approaches with existing cognitive-behavioral models. *Clinical Psychology: Science and Practice, 9,* 54–68. doi:10.1093/clipsy.9.1.54

Roemer, L., Orsillo, S. M., & Salters-Pedneault, K. (2008). Efficacy of an acceptance-based behavior therapy for generalized anxiety disorder: Evaluation in a randomized controlled trial. *Journal of Consulting and Clinical Psychology, 76,* 1083–1089. doi:10.1037/a0012720

Segal, Z. V., Williams, M. G., & Teasdale, J. D. (2001). *Mindfulness-based cognitive therapy for depression: A new approach to preventing relapse* (1st ed.). New York, NY: Guilford Press.

Stanley, M. A., Wilson, N. L., Novy, D. M., Rhoades, H. M., Wagener, P. D., Greisinger, A. J., ... Kunik, M. E. (2009). Cognitive behavior therapy for generalized anxiety disorder among older adults in primary care: A randomized clinical trial. *JAMA, 301,* 1460–1467. doi:10.1001/jama.2009.458

Starcevic, B., & Bogojevic, G. (1999). The concept of generalized anxiety disorder: Between the too narrow and too wide diagnostic criteria. *Psychopathology, 32,* 5–11.

Stober, J. (1998). Reliability and validity of two widely-used worry questionnaires: Self-report and self-peer convergence. *Personality and Individual Differences, 24,* 887–890.

Tallis, F., Eysenck, M.W., & Mathews, A. (1992). A questionnaire for the measurement of nonpathological worry. *Personality and Individual Differences, 13,* 161–168.

Vrana, S. R., Cuthbert, B. N., & Lang, P. J. (1986). Fear imagery and text processing. *Psychophysiology, 23,* 247–253.

Warshaw, M. G., Keller, M. B., & Stout, R. L. (1994). Reliability and validity of the longitudinal interval follow-up evaluation for assessing outcome of anxiety disorders. *Journal of Psychiatric Research, 28,* 531–545.

Waters, A. M., & Craske, M. G. (2005). *Generalized anxiety disorder.* New York, NY: Guildford Press.

Wells, A. (2005). The metacognitive model of GAD: Assessment of meta-worry and relationship with DSM-IV generalized anxiety disorder. *Cognitive Therapy and Research, 29*(1), 107–121. doi:10.1007/s10608-005-1652-0

Wells, A., & King, P. (2006). Metacognitive therapy for generalized anxiety disorder: An open trial. *Journal of Behavior Therapy and Experimental Psychiatry, 37,* 206–212.

Wittchen, H.-U., Zhao, S., Kessler, R. C., & Eaton, W. W. (1994). DSM-II-R generalized anxiety disorder in the National Comorbidity Survey. *Archives of General Psychiatry, 51,* 355–364.

World Health Organization. (1992). *ICD-10: The ICD-10 classification of mental and behavioural disorders: Clinical descriptions and diagnostic guidelines.* Geneva: Author.

Yonkers, K. A., Massion, A., Warshaw, M., & Keller, M. B. (1996). Phenomenology and course of generalized anxiety disorder. *British Journal of Psychiatry, 168,* 308–313.

Zimmerman, M., & Mattia, J. I. (2001a). The psychiatric diagnostic screening questionnaire: Development, reliability and validity. *Comprehensive Psychiatry, 42,* 175–189. doi:10.1053/comp.2001.23126

Zimmerman, M., & Mattia, J. I. (2001b). A self-report scale to help make psychiatric diagnoses: The Psychiatric Diagnostic Screening Questionnaire. *Arch Gen Psychiatry, 58,* 787–794. doi:10.1001/archpsyc.58.8.787

Zinbarg, R. E., Craske, M. G., & Barlow, D. H. (2006). *Mastery of your anxiety and worry (MAW): Therapist guide* (2nd ed.). New York, NY: Oxford University Press.

8

Appendix: Tools and Resources

Appendix 1: Penn State Worry Questionnaire (PSWQ)
Appendix 2: Worry Domains Questionnaire (WDQ)
Appendix 3: Why Worry Questionnaire (WW-II)
Appendix 4: Consequences of Worry (COWS)
Appendix 5: The Acceptance and Action Questionnaire (AAQ-II)
Appendix 6: Intolerance of Uncertainty Scale (IUS)
Appendix 7: Depression, Anxiety, and Stress Scale (DASS-21)
Appendix 8: Meta-Worry Questionnaire (MWQ)
Appendix 9: Worry and Anxiety Questionnaire (WAQ)
Appendix 10: Case Conceptualization Form for Client
Appendix 11: Intolerance of Uncertainty Monitoring Form
Appendix 12: Example of Pie Chart Representing Valued Areas

Penn State Worry Questionnaire (PSWQ)

Enter the number that best describes how typical or characteristic each item is of you, putting the number next to the item.

1	2	3	4	5
Not at all typical		Somewhat typical		Very typical

1. _____ If I don't have enough time to do everything, I don't worry about it.

2. _____ My worries overwhelm me.

3. _____ I do not tend to worry about things.

4. _____ Many situations make me worry.

5. _____ I know I shouldn't worry about things, but I just cannot help it.

6. _____ When I am under pressure I worry a lot.

7. _____ I am always worrying about something.

8. _____ I find it easy to dismiss worrisome thoughts.

9. _____ As soon as I finish one task, I start to worry about everything else I have to do.

10. _____ I never worry about anything

11. _____ When there is nothing more I can do about a concern, I don't worry about it anymore.

12. _____ I've been a worrier all my life.

13. _____ I notice that I have been worrying about things.

14. _____ Once I start worrying, I can't stop.

15. _____ I worry all the time.

16. _____ I worry about projects until they are done.

Reprinted from *Behavior Research and Therapy, 28,* T. J. Meyer, M. L. Miller, R. L. Metzger, and T. D. Borkovec, "Development and validation of the Penn State Worry Questionnaire," 487–495, Copyright (1990) with permission from Elsevier.

Worry Domains Questionnaire (WDQ)

Please indicate, by circling the appropriate number, how much you think each of the following statements describes YOU when you worry.

1 = Not at all
2 = A little
3 = Moderately
4 = Quite a bit
5 = Extremely

I worry...

1. that my money will run out

    1   2   3   4   5

2. that I cannot be assertive or express my opinions

    1   2   3   4   5

3. that my future job prospects are not good

    1   2   3   4   5

4. that my family will be angry with me or disapprove of something that I do

    1   2   3   4   5

5. that I'll never achieve my ambitions

    1   2   3   4   5

6. that I will not keep my workload up to date

    1   2   3   4   5

7. that financial problems will restrict holidays and travel

    1   2   3   4   5

8. that I have no concentration

    1   2   3   4   5

9. that I am not able to afford things

    1   2   3   4   5

10. that I feel insecure

    1   2   3   4   5

11. that I can't afford to pay my bills

    1   2   3   4   5

12. that my living conditions are inadequate

    1   2   3   4   5

13. that life may have no purpose

    1   2   3   4   5

14. that I don't work hard enough

| 1 | 2 | 3 | 4 | 5 |

15. that others will not approve of me

| 1 | 2 | 3 | 4 | 5 |

16. that I find it difficult to maintain a stable relationship

| 1 | 2 | 3 | 4 | 5 |

17. that I leave work unfinished

| 1 | 2 | 3 | 4 | 5 |

18. that I lack confidence

| 1 | 2 | 3 | 4 | 5 |

19. that I am unattractive

| 1 | 2 | 3 | 4 | 5 |

20. that I might make myself look stupid

| 1 | 2 | 3 | 4 | 5 |

21. that I will lose close friends

| 1 | 2 | 3 | 4 | 5 |

22. that I haven't achieved much

| 1 | 2 | 3 | 4 | 5 |

23. that I am not loved

| 1 | 2 | 3 | 4 | 5 |

24. that I will be late for an appointment

| 1 | 2 | 3 | 4 | 5 |

25. that I make mistakes at work

| 1 | 2 | 3 | 4 | 5 |

Why Worry Questionnaire (WW-II)

Below are a series of statements that can be related to worry. Please think back to times when you are worried and indicate by circling a number (0 to 5), to what extent these statements are true for you.

1 = Not at all true
2 = Slightly true
3 = Somewhat true
4 = Very true
5 = Absolutely true

1. If I did not worry, I would be careless and irresponsible.
      1   2   3   4   5

2. If I worry, I will be less disturbed when unforeseen events occur.
      1   2   3   4   5

3. I worry in order to know what to do.
      1   2   3   4   5

4. If I worry in advance, I will be less disappointed if something serious occurs.
      1   2   3   4   5

5. The fact that I worry helps me plan my actions to solve a problem.
      1   2   3   4   5

6. The act of worrying itself can prevent mishaps from occurring.
      1   2   3   4   5

7. If I did not worry, it would make me a negligent person.
      1   2   3   4   5

8. It is by worrying that I finally undertake the work that I must do.
      1   2   3   4   5

9. I worry because I think it can help me find a solution to my problem.
      1   2   3   4   5

10. The fact that I worry shows that I am a person who takes care of their affairs.
       1   2   3   4   5

11. Thinking too much about positive things can prevent them from occurring.
       1   2   3   4   5

12. The fact that I worry confirms that I am a prudent person.
       1   2   3   4   5

13. If misfortune comes, I will feel less responsible if I have been worrying about it beforehand.
       1   2   3   4   5

14. By worrying I can find a better way to do things.
       1   2   3   4   5

15. Worrying stimulates me and makes me more effective.

    1   2   3   4   5

16. The fact that I worry incites me to act.

    1   2   3   4   5

17. The act of worrying itself reduces the risk that something serious will occur.

    1   2   3   4   5

18. By worrying I do certain things, which I would not decide to do otherwise.

    1   2   3   4   5

19. The fact that I worry motivates me to do the things I must do.

    1   2   3   4   5

20. My worries can, by themselves, reduces the risks of danger.

    1   2   3   4   5

21. If I worry less, I decrease my chances of finding the best solution.

    1   2   3   4   5

22. The fact that I worry will allow me to feel less guilty if something serious occurs.

    1   2   3   4   5

23. If I worry, I will be less unhappy when a negative event occurs.

    1   2   3   4   5

24. By not worrying, one can attract misfortune.

    1   2   3   4   5

25. The fact that I worry shows that I am a good person.

    1   2   3   4   5

Consequences of Worry (COWS)

Please indicate, by circling the appropriate number, how much you think each of the following state-ments describes YOU when you worry.

1 = Not at all
2 = A little
3 = Moderately
4 = Quite a bit
5 = A lot

1. Worrying distorts the problem I have, so I am unable to solve it.
    1   2   3   4   5

2. By worrying, I reorganize and plan my time better – if I stick to it, it makes me feel better.
    1   2   3   4   5

3. Worrying starts off as a process of preparing me to meet new situations.
    1   2   3   4   5

4. Worrying makes me depressed and therefore makes it harder to concentrate and get on with things.
    1   2   3   4   5

5. When I worry, it stops me from taking decisive action.
    1   2   3   4   5

6. Worrying weakens me by affecting my levels of energy in response to those events that worry me.
    1   2   3   4   5

7. Working makes me tense and irritable.
    1   2   3   4   5

8. Worrying clarifies my thoughts and concentration.
    1   2   3   4   5

9. Worrying acts as a stimulant.
    1   2   3   4   5

10. Worrying causes me stress.
    1   2   3   4   5

11. Worrying stops me dealing with certain situations.
    1   2   3   4   5

12. Worrying makes me irrational.
    1   2   3   4   5

13. Worrying challenges and motivates me, without it I would not achieve much in life.
    1   2   3   4   5

14. Worrying gets me worked up.
    1   2   3   4   5

15. Deep down I know I do not need to worry that much, but I can't help it.

     1   2   3   4   5

16. Worrying increases my anxiety and so decreases my performance.

     1   2   3   4   5

17. Worrying gives me the opportunity to analyze situations and work out the pros and cons.

     1   2   3   4   5

18. Problems are magnified when I dwell on them.

     1   2   3   4   5

19. Worrying increases my anxiety.

     1   2   3   4   5

20. Worrying stops me from thinking straight.

     1   2   3   4   5

21. Worrying allows me to work through the worst that can happen, so when it doesn't happen, things are better.

     1   2   3   4   5

22. Worrying makes me do things by increasing my adrenalin levels.

     1   2   3   4   5

23. Worry makes me focus on the wrong things.

     1   2   3   4   5

24. In order to get something done, I have to worry about it.

     1   2   3   4   5

25. Worrying makes me reflect on life by asking questions I might not usually ask when happy.

     1   2   3   4   5

26. I become paranoid when I worry.

     1   2   3   4   5

27. Worrying gives me a pessimistic and fatalistic outlook.

     1   2   3   4   5

28. Worrying adds concern to the problem and as such leads me to explore different possibilities.

     1   2   3   4   5

29. Worrying increases my awareness, thus increasing my performance.

     1   2   3   4   5

The Acceptance and Action Questionnaire (AAQ-II)

Below you will find a list of statements. Please rate how true each statement is for you by circling a number next to it. Use the scale below to make your choice.

1 = Never true
2 = Very seldom true
3 = Seldom true
4 = Sometimes true
5 = Frequently true
6 = Almost always true
7 = Always true

1. It's OK if I remember something unpleasant.

    1   2   3   4   5

2. My painful experiences and memories make it difficult for me to live a life that I would value.

    1   2   3   4   5

3. I'm afraid of my feelings.

    1   2   3   4   5

4. I worry about not being able to control my worries and feelings.

    1   2   3   4   5

5. My painful memories prevent me from having a fulfilling life.

    1   2   3   4   5

6. I am in control of my life.

    1   2   3   4   5

7. Emotions cause problems in my life.

    1   2   3   4   5

8. It seems like most people are handling their lives better than I am.

    1   2   3   4   5

9. Worries get in the way of my success.

    1   2   3   4   5

10. My thoughts and feelings do not get in the way of how I want to live my life.

    1   2   3   4   5

Intolerance of Uncertainty Scale (IUS)

You will find below a series of statements which describe how people may react to the uncertainties of life. Please use the scale below to describe to what extent each item is characteristic of you. Please circle a number (1 to 5) that describes you best.

1	2	3	4	5
Not at all characteristic of me		Somewhat characteristic of me		Entirely characteristic of me

1. Uncertain stops me from having a firm opinion.

    1   2   3   4   5

2. Being uncertain means that a person is disorganized.

    1   2   3   4   5

3. Uncertainty makes life intolerable.

    1   2   3   4   5

4. It's unfair not having any guarantees in life.

    1   2   3   4   5

5. My mind can't be relaxed if I don't know what will happen tomorrow.

    1   2   3   4   5

6. Uncertainty makes me uneasy, anxious, or stressed.

    1   2   3   4   5

7. Unforeseen events upset me greatly.

    1   2   3   4   5

8. It frustrates me not having all the information I need.

    1   2   3   4   5

9. Uncertainty keeps me from living a full life.

    1   2   3   4   5

10. One should always look ahead so as to avoid surprises.

    1   2   3   4   5

11. A small unforeseen event can spoil everything, even with the best of planning.

    1   2   3   4   5

12. When it's time to act, uncertainty paralyses me.

    1   2   3   4   5

13. Being uncertain means that I am not first rate.

    1   2   3   4   5

14. When I am uncertain, I can't go forward.

    1   2   3   4   5

15. When I am uncertain, I can't function very well.

    1   2   3   4   5

16. Unlike me, others always seem to know where they are going with their lives.

    1   2   3   4   5

17. Uncertainty makes me vulnerable, unhappy, or sad.

    1   2   3   4   5

18. I always want to know what the future has in store for me.

    1   2   3   4   5

19. I can't stand being taken by surprise.

    1   2   3   4   5

20. The smallest doubt can stop me from acting.

    1   2   3   4   5

21. I should be able to organize everything in advance.

    1   2   3   4   5

22. Being uncertain means that I lack confidence.

    1   2   3   4   5

23. I think it's unfair that other people seem sure about their future.

    1   2   3   4   5

24. Uncertainty keeps me from sleeping soundly.

    1   2   3   4   5

25. I must get away from all uncertain situations.

    1   2   3   4   5

26. The ambiguities in life stress me.

    1   2   3   4   5

27. I can't stand being undecided about my future.

    1   2   3   4   5

Depression, Anxiety, and Stress Scale (DASS-21)

Please read each statement and circle a number 0, 1, 2 or 3 that indicates how much the statement applied to you *over the past week*. There are no right or wrong answers. Do not spend too much time on any statement.

0 = Did not apply to me at all
1 = Applied to me to some degree, or some of the time
2 = Applied to me to a considerable degree, or a good part of time
3 = Applied to me very much, or most of the time

1.   I found it hard to wind down.

     0   1   2   3

2.   I was aware of dryness of my mouth.

     0   1   2   3

3.   I couldn't seem to experience any positive feeling at all.

     0   1   2   3

4.   I experienced breathing difficulty (e.g., excessively rapid breathing, breathlessness in the absence of physical exertion).

     0   1   2   3

5.   I found it difficult to work up the initiative to do things.

     0   1   2   3

6.   I tended to over-react to situations.

     0   1   2   3

7.   I experienced trembling (e.g., in the hands).

     0   1   2   3

8.   I felt that I was using a lot of nervous energy.

     0   1   2   3

9.   I was worried about situations in which I might panic and make a fool of myself.

     0   1   2   3

10. I felt that I had nothing to look forward to.

     0   1   2   3

11. I found myself getting agitated.

     0   1   2   3

12. I found it difficult to relax.

     0   1   2   3

13. I felt down-hearted and blue.

     0   1   2   3

14. I was intolerant of anything that kept me from getting on with what I was doing.

    0   1   2   3

15. I felt I was close to panic.

    0   1   2   3

16. I was unable to become enthusiastic about anything.

    0   1   2   3

17. I felt I wasn't worth much as a person.

    0   1   2   3

18. I felt that I was rather touchy.

    0   1   2   3

19. I was aware of the action of my heart in the absence of physical exertion (e.g., sense of heart rate increase, heart missing a beat).

    0   1   2   3

20. I felt scared without any good reason.

    0   1   2   3

21. I felt that life was meaningless.

    0   1   2   3

The DASS-21 is in the public domain and may be downloaded from www.psy.unsw.edu.au/dass/

Meta-Worry Questionnaire (MWQ)

Please read each statement and circle a number 1, 2, 3, or 4 that indicates how much the statement applies to you. There are no right or wrong answers. Do not spend too much time on any statement.

1 = Never
2 = Sometimes
3 = Often
4 = Almost always

1. I am going crazy with worrying.

     1   2   3   4

2. My worrying will escalate and I'll cease to function.

     1   2   3   4

3. I'm making myself ill with worry.

     1   2   3   4

4. I'm abnormal for worrying.

     1   2   3   4

5. My mind can't take the worrying.

     1   2   3   4

6. I'm losing out in life because of worrying.

     1   2   3   4

7. My body can't take the worrying

     1   2   3   4

Worry and Anxiety Questionnaire (WAQ)

1. What subjects do you worry about most often?

a. _____

b. _____

c. _____

d. _____

e. _____

For the following items, please circle the corresponding number (0–8)

2. Do your worries seem excessive or exaggerated?

Not at all Excessive				Moderately excessive				Totally excessive
0	1	2	3	4	5	6	7	8

3. Over the past 6 months, how many days have you been bothered by excessive worry?

Never				1 day out of 2				Every day
0	1	2	3	4	5	6	7	8

4. Do you have difficulty controlling your worries? For example, when you start worrying about something, do you have difficulty stopping?

No difficulty				Moderate difficulty				Extreme difficulty
0	1	2	3	4	5	6	7	8

5. Over the past 6 months, to what extent have you been disturbed by the following sensations when you were worried or anxious?

a. Restlessness or feeling keyed up or on edge.

Not at all				Moderately				Very Severely
0	1	2	3	4	5	6	7	8

b. Being easily fatigued.

Not at all				Moderately				Very Severely
0	1	2	3	4	5	6	7	8

c. Difficulty concentrating or mind going blank.

Not at all				Moderately				Very Severely
0	1	2	3	4	5	6	7	8

d. Irritability.

Not at all				Moderately				Very Severely
0	1	2	3	4	5	6	7	8

e. Muscle tension.

Not at all				Moderately				Very Severely
0	1	2	3	4	5	6	7	8

f. Sleep disturbance (difficulty falling or staying asleep, or restless unsatisfying sleep).

Not at all				Moderately				Very Severely
0	1	2	3	4	5	6	7	8

6. To what extent does worry or anxiety interfere with your life? For example, your work, social activities, family life, etc.?

Not at all				Moderately				Very Severely
0	1	2	3	4	5	6	7	8

Case Conceptualization Form for Client

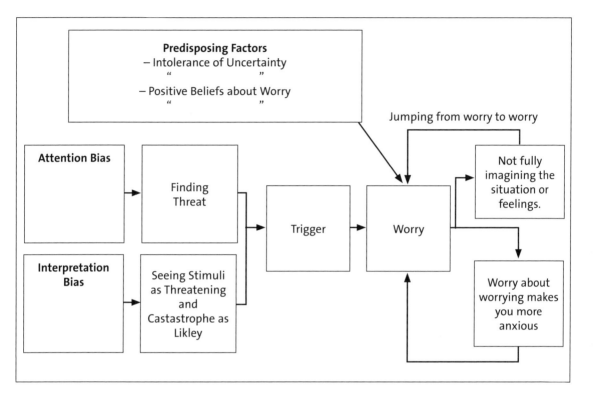

Intolerance of Uncertainty Monitoring Form

Date: _____

Trigger for worry (What do you remember happening before the worry started?): _____

_____

_____

_____

Thoughts associated with the worry: _____

_____

_____

_____

Was worry used to reduce uncertainty? Explain: _____

_____

_____

_____

Other behaviors engaged in because of worry (What did the worry make you want to do?):

_____

_____

_____

Duration of worry: _____

From: C. D. Marker and A. G. Aylward: *Generalized Anxiety Disorder*   © 2012 Hogrefe Publishing

Example of Pie Chart Representing Valued Areas

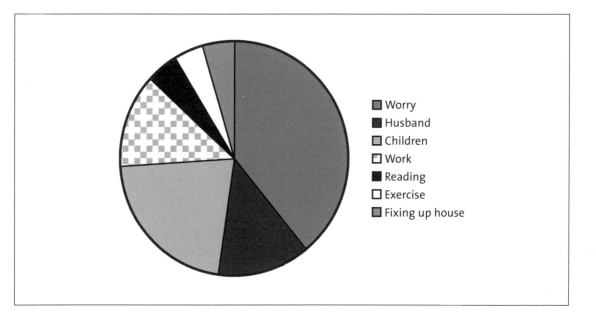

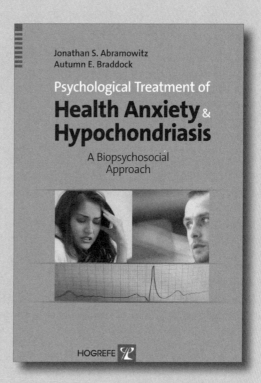
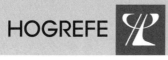

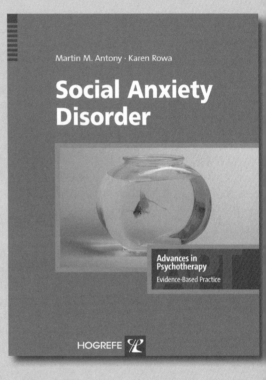 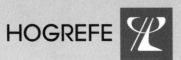

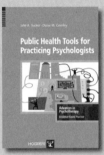
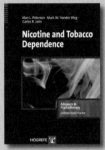
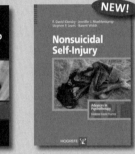
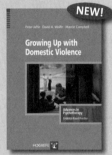
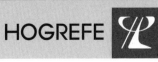

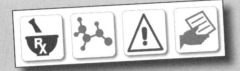
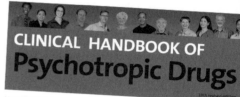

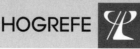